Virtual Clinical Excursions—General Hospital

for

Potter, Perry, Stockert, and Hall:
Fundamentals of Nursing,
Eighth Edition

Virtual Clinical Excursions—General Hospital

for

Potter, Perry, Stockert, and Hall:
Fundamentals of Nursing,
Eighth Edition

prepared by

Kim D. Cooper, RN, MSN
Ivy Tech Community College
Terre Haute, Indiana

software developed by

Wolfsong Informatics, LLC
Tucson, Arizona

3251 Riverport Lane
Maryland Heights, Missouri 63043

VIRTUAL CLINICAL EXCURSIONS—GENERAL HOSPITAL FOR
POTTER, PERRY, STOCKERT, AND HALL: FUNDAMENTALS OF NURSING,
EIGHTH EDITION

ISBN: 978-0-323-08867-1

Copyright © 2013 by Mosby, an imprint of Elsevier Inc.
Copyright © 2009 by Mosby, Inc., an affiliate of Elsevier Inc.

Notice

Knowledge and best practice in this field are constantly changing. As new research and experience broaden our understanding, changes in research methods, professional practices, or medical treatment may become necessary.

Practitioners and researchers must always rely on their own experience and knowledge in evaluating and using any information, methods, compounds, or experiments described herein. In using such information or methods they should be mindful of their own safety and the safety of others, including parties for whom they have a professional responsibility.

With respect to any drug or pharmaceutical products identified, readers are advised to check the most current information provided (i) on procedures featured or (ii) by the manufacturer of each product to be administered, to verify the recommended dose or formula, the method and duration of administration, and contraindications. It is the responsibility of practitioners, relying on their own experience and knowledge of their patients, to make diagnoses, to determine dosages and the best treatment for each individual patient, and to take all appropriate safety precautions.

To the fullest extent of the law, neither the Publisher nor the authors, contributors, or editors, assume any liability for any injury and/or damage to persons or property as a matter of products liability, negligence or otherwise, or from any use or operation of any methods, products, instructions, or ideas contained in the material herein.

ISBN: 978-0-323-08867-1

Vice President eSolutions—Nursing: *Tom Wilhelm*
Director, Simulation Solutions: *Jeff Downing*
Associate Content Development Specialist: *Krissy Prysmiki*
Publishing Services Manager: *Jeffery Patterson*
Senior Project Manager: *Tracey Schriefer*

Printed in the United States of America

Last digit is the print number: 9 8 7 6 5 4 3

Workbook
prepared by

Kim D. Cooper, RN, MSN
Ivy Tech Community College
Terre Haute, Indiana

Textbook

Patricia A. Potter, RN, PhD, FAAN
Director of Research, Patient Care Services
Barnes-Jewish Hospital
St. Louis, Missouri

Anne Griffin Perry, RN, EdD, FAAN
Professor and Associate Dean
School of Nursing
Southern Illinois University Edwardsville
Edwardsville, Illinois

Patricia Stockert, RN, BSN, MS, PhD
President of the College
Saint Francis Medical Center College of Nursing
Peoria, Illinois

Amy Hall, RN, BSN, MS, PhD, CNE
Chair and White Family Endowed Professor of Nursing
Dunigan Family Department of Nursing and Health Sciences
University of Evansville
Evansville, Indiana

Table of Contents
Virtual Clinical Excursions Workbook

Table of Contents
Potter and Perry
Fundamentals of Nursing, Eighth Edition

Unit 6—Psychosocial Basis for Nursing Practice

Unit 7—Physiological Basis for Nursing Practice

Getting Started

GETTING SET UP WITH VCE ONLINE

The product you have purchased is part of the Evolve Learning System. Please read the following information thoroughly to get started.

■ HOW TO ACCESS YOUR VCE RESOURCES ON EVOLVE

There are two ways to access your VCE Resources on Evolve:

1. If your instructor has enrolled you into your VCE Evolve Resources you will receive an email with your registration details.

2. If your instructor has asked you to self-enroll into your VCE Evolve Resources they will provide you with your Course ID (for example: 1479_jdoe73_0001). You will then need to follow the instructions at https://evolve.elsevier.com/cs/studentEnroll.html.

There are two ways to access the virtual hospital portion of *Virtual Clinical Excursions:* online through the Evolve VCE Resources or via the CD-ROM that accompanies the VCE workbook. Instructions for both are provided below.

■ HOW TO ACCESS THE ONLINE VIRTUAL HOSPITAL

The online virtual hospital is available through the Evolve VCE Resources. There is no software to download or install: the online virtual hospital runs within your internet browser, using a popup window.

ONLINE: TECHNICAL REQUIREMENTS

*   Broadband connection (DSL or cable)
*   1024 x 768 screen resolution
*   Mozilla Firefox 18.0, Internet Explorer 9.0, Google Chrome and Safari 5 or higher
    Note: Pop-up blocking software/settings must be disabled.
*   Adobe Acrobat Reader
*   Additional technical requirements can be found at http://evolvesupport.elsevier.com.

■ HOW TO ACCESS THE VIRTUAL HOSPITAL VIA THE CD-ROM

The virtual hospital is available through the CD-ROM located in the back of your print workbook.

CD-ROM: MINIMUM SYSTEM REQUIREMENTS

WINDOWS®

Windows Vista®, XP, 2000 (Recommend Windows XP/2000)
Pentium® III processor (or equivalent) @ 600 MHz (Recommend 800 MHz or better)
256 MB of RAM (Recommend 1 GB or more for Windows Vista)
800 x 600 screen size (Recommend 1024 x 768)
Thousands of colors
12x CD-ROM drive

Note: Windows Vista and XP require administrator privileges for installation.

MACINTOSH® (*Note:* This CD will not work in Mac Lion 10.7)

MAC OS X (up to 10.6)
Apple Power PC G3 @ 500 MHz or better
128 MB of RAM (Recommend 256 MB or more)
800 x 600 screen size (Recommend 1024 x 768)
Thousands of colors
12x CD-ROM drive
Stereo speakers or headphones

CD-ROM: INSTALLATION INSTRUCTIONS

WINDOWS

1. Insert the *Virtual Clinical Excursions* CD-ROM.
2. The setup screen should appear automatically if the current product is not already installed. Windows Vista users may be asked to authorize additional security prompts.
3. Follow the onscreen instructions during the setup process.

    If the setup screen does *not* appear automatically (and *Virtual Clinical Excursions* has not been installed already):
    a. Click the **My Computer** icon on your desktop or on your Start menu.
    b. Double-click on your CD-ROM drive.
    c. If installation does not start at this point:
        (1) Click the **Start** icon on the taskbar and select the **Run** option.
        (2) Type d:\setup.exe (where "d:\" is your CD-ROM drive) and press **OK**.
        (3) Follow the onscreen instructions for installation.

MACINTOSH

1. Insert the *Virtual Clinical Excursions* CD in the CD-ROM drive. The disk icon will appear on your desktop.
2. Double-click on the disk icon.
3. Double-click on the MAC run file.

Note: Virtual Clinical Excursions for Macintosh does not have an installation setup and can only be run directly from the CD.

CD-ROM: HOW TO USE VIRTUAL CLINICAL EXCURSIONS

WINDOWS

1. Double-click on the *Virtual Clinical Excursions* icon located on your desktop.
2. Or navigate to the program via the Windows Start menu.

Note: If your computer uses Windows Vista, right-click on the desktop shortcut and choose **Properties**. In the Compatibility Mode, check the box for "Run as Administrator."

MACINTOSH

1. Insert the *Virtual Clinical Excursions* CD in the CD-ROM drive. The disk icon will appear on your desktop.
2. Double-click on the disk icon.
3. Double-click on the MAC run file.

■ HOW TO ACCESS THE WORKBOOK

There are two ways to access the workbook portion of *Virtual Clinical Excursions:*

1. Print workbook
2. An electronic version of the workbook is available within the VCE Evolve Resources.

■ TECHNICAL SUPPORT

Technical support for *Virtual Clinical Excursions* is available by visiting the Technical Support Center at http://evolvesupport.elsevier.com or by calling 1-800-222-9570 inside the United States and Canada.

Trademarks: Windows® and Macintosh® are registered trademarks.

A QUICK TOUR

Welcome to *Virtual Clinical Excursions—General Hospital*, a virtual hospital setting in which you can work with multiple complex patient simulations and also learn to access and evaluate the information resources that are essential for high-quality patient care. The virtual hospital, Pacific View Regional Hospital, has realistic architecture and access to patient rooms, a Nurses' Station, and a Medication Room.

■ BEFORE YOU START

Make sure you have your textbook nearby when you use *Virtual Clinical Excursions*. You will want to consult topic areas in your textbook frequently while working with the virtual hospital and workbook.

■ HOW TO SIGN IN

- Enter your name on the Student Nurse identification badge.
- Next, specify the floor on which you will work by clicking the down arrow next to **Select Floor**. For this quick tour, choose **Medical-Surgical**.
- Now click the down arrow next to **Select Period of Care**. This drop-down menu gives you four periods of care from which to choose. In Periods of Care 1 through 3, you can actively engage in patient assessment, entry of data in the electronic patient record (EPR), and medication administration. Period of Care 4 presents the day in review. Highlight and click the appropriate period of care. (For this quick tour, choose **Period of Care 1: 0730-0815**.)
- Click **Go**. This takes you to the Patient List screen (see the How to Select a Patient section below). Note that the virtual time is provided in the box at the lower left corner of the screen (0730, since we chose Period of Care 1).

Note: If you choose to work during Period of Care 4: 1900-2000, the Patient List screen is skipped since you are not able to visit patients or administer medications during the shift. Instead, you are taken directly to the Nurses' Station, where the records of all the patients on the floor are available for your review.

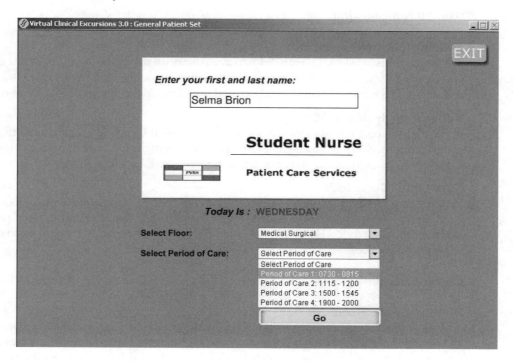

■ PATIENT LIST

MEDICAL-SURGICAL UNIT

Harry George (Room 401)
Osteomyelitis—A 54-year-old Caucasian male admitted from a homeless shelter with an infected leg. He has complications of type 2 diabetes mellitus, alcohol abuse, nicotine addiction, poor pain control, and complex psychosocial issues.

Jacquline Catanazaro (Room 402)
Asthma—A 45-year-old Caucasian female admitted with an acute asthma exacerbation and suspected pneumonia. She has complications of chronic schizophrenia, noncompliance with medication therapy, obesity, and herniated disc.

Piya Jordan (Room 403)
Bowel obstruction—A 68-year-old Asian female admitted with a colon mass and suspected adenocarcinoma. She undergoes a right hemicolectomy. This patient's complications include atrial fibrillation, hypokalemia, and symptoms of meperidine toxicity.

Clarence Hughes (Room 404)
Degenerative joint disease—A 73-year-old African-American male admitted for a left total knee replacement. His preparations for discharge are complicated by the development of a pulmonary embolus and the need for ongoing intravenous therapy.

Pablo Rodriguez (Room 405)
Metastatic lung carcinoma—A 71-year-old Hispanic male admitted with symptoms of dehydration and malnutrition. He has chronic pain secondary to multiple subcutaneous skin nodules and psychosocial concerns related to family issues with his approaching death.

Patricia Newman (Room 406)
Pneumonia—A 61-year-old Caucasian female admitted with worsening pulmonary function and an acute respiratory infection. Her chronic emphysema is complicated by heavy smoking, hypertension, and malnutrition. She needs access to community resources such as a smoking cessation program and meal assistance.

SKILLED NURSING UNIT

William Jefferson (Room 501)
Alzheimer's disease—A 75-year-old African-American male admitted for stabilization of type 2 diabetes and hypertension following a recent acute care admission for a urinary tract infection and sepsis. His complications include episodes of acute delirium and a history of osteoarthritis.

Kathryn Doyle (Room 503)
Rehabilitation post left hip replacement—A 79-year-old Caucasian female admitted following a complicated recovery from an ORIF. She is experiencing symptoms of malnutrition and depression due to unstable family dynamics, placing her at risk for elder abuse.

Goro Oishi (Room 505)
Hospice care—A 66-year-old Asian male admitted following an acute care admission for an intracerebral hemorrhage and resulting coma. Family-staff interactions provide opportunities to explore death and dying issues related to conflict about advanced life support and cultural and religious differences.

OBSTETRICS UNIT

Dorothy Grant (Room 201)
30-week intrauterine pregnancy—A 25-year-old multipara Caucasian female admitted with abdominal trauma following a domestic violence incident. Her complications include preterm labor and extensive social issues such as acquiring safe housing for her family upon discharge.

■ HOW TO SELECT A PATIENT

- You can choose one or more patients to work with from the Patient List by checking the box to the left of the patient name(s). For this quick tour, select Piya Jordan and Pablo Rodriguez. (In order to receive a scorecard for a patient, the patient must be selected before proceeding to the Nurses' Station.)
- Click on **Get Report** to the right of the medical records number (MRN) to view a summary of the patient's care during the 12-hour period before your arrival on the unit.
- After reviewing the report, click on **Go to Nurses' Station** in the right lower corner to begin your care. (*Note:* If you have been assigned to care for multiple patients, you can click on **Return to Patient List** to select and review the report for each additional patient before going to the Nurses' Station.)

Note: Even though the Patient List is initially skipped when you sign in to work for Period of Care 4, you can still access this screen if you wish to review the shift report for any of the patients. To do so, simply click on **Patient List** near the top left corner of the Nurses' Station (or click on the clipboard to the left of the Kardex). Then click on **Get Report** for the patient(s) whose care you are reviewing. This may be done during any period of care.

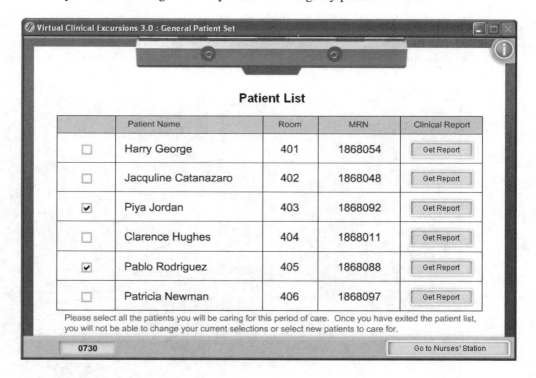

■ HOW TO FIND A PATIENT'S RECORDS

NURSES' STATION

Within the Nurses' Station, you will see:

1. A clipboard that contains the patient list for that floor.
2. A chart rack with patient charts labeled by room number, a notebook labeled Kardex, and a notebook labeled MAR (Medication Administration Record).
3. A desktop computer with access to the Electronic Patient Record (EPR).
4. A tool bar across the top of the screen that can also be used to access the Patient List, EPR, Chart, MAR, and Kardex. This tool bar is also accessible from each patient's room.
5. A Drug Guide containing information about the medications you are able to administer to your patients.
6. A Laboratory Guide containing normal value ranges for all laboratory tests you may come across in the virtual patient hospital.
7. A tool bar across the bottom of the screen that can be used to access the Floor Map, patient rooms, Medication Room, and Drug Guide.

As you run your cursor over an item, it will be highlighted. To select, simply click on the item. As you use these resources, you will always be able to return to the Nurses' Station by clicking on the **Return to Nurses' Station** bar located in the right lower corner of your screen.

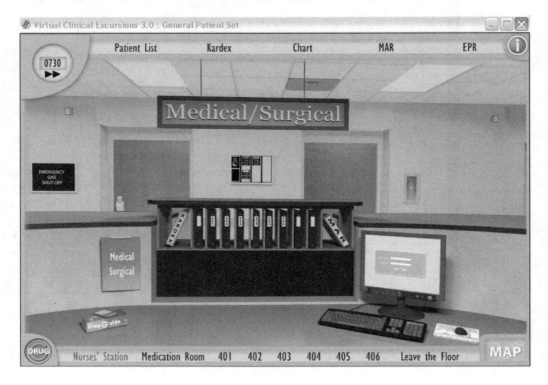

MEDICATION ADMINISTRATION RECORD (MAR)

The MAR icon located on the tool bar at the top of your screen accesses current 24-hour medications for each patient. Click on the icon and the MAR will open. (*Note:* You can also access the MAR by clicking on the MAR notebook on the far right side of the book rack in the center of the screen.) Within the MAR, tabs on the right side of the screen allow you to select patients by room number. Be careful to make sure you select the correct tab number for *your* patient rather than simply reading the first record that appears after the MAR opens. Each MAR sheet lists the following:

- Medications
- Route and dosage of each medication
- Times of administration of each medication

Note: The MAR changes each day. Expired MARs are stored in the patients' charts.

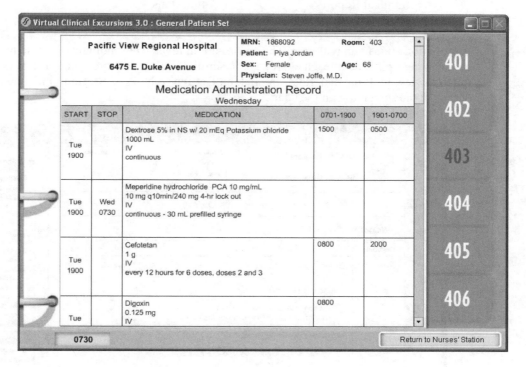

Charts

To access patient charts, either click on the **Chart** icon at the top of your screen or anywhere within the chart rack in the center of the Nurses' Station screen. When the close-up view appears, the individual charts are labeled by room number. To open a chart, click on the room number of the patient whose chart you wish to review. The patient's name and allergies will appear on the left side of the screen, along with a list of tabs on the right side of the screen, allowing you to view the following data:

- Allergies
- Physician's Orders
- Physician's Notes
- Nurse's Notes
- Laboratory Reports
- Diagnostic Reports
- Surgical Reports
- Consultations

- Patient Education
- History and Physical
- Nursing Admission
- Expired MARs
- Consents
- Mental Health
- Admissions
- Emergency Department

Information appears in real time. The entries are in reverse chronologic order, so use the down arrow at the right side of each chart page to scroll down to view previous entries. Flip from tab to tab to view multiple data fields or click on **Return to Nurses' Station** in the lower right corner of the screen to exit the chart.

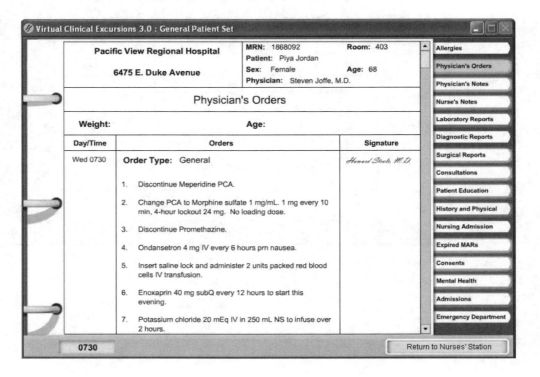

ELECTRONIC PATIENT RECORD (EPR)

The EPR can be accessed from the computer in the Nurses' Station or from the EPR icon located in the tool bar at the top of your screen. To access a patient's EPR:
- Click on either the computer screen or the **EPR** icon.
- Your username and password are automatically filled in.
- Click on **Login** to enter the EPR.
- *Note:* Like the MAR, the EPR is arranged numerically. Thus when you enter, you are initially shown the records of the patient in the lowest room number on the floor. To view the correct data for *your* patient, remember to select the correct room number, using the drop-down menu for the Patient field at the top left corner of the screen.

The EPR used in Pacific View Regional Hospital represents a composite of commercial versions being used in hospitals. You can access the EPR:
- to review existing data for a patient (by room number).
- to enter data you collect while working with a patient.

The EPR is updated daily, so no matter what day or part of a shift you are working, there will be a current EPR with the patient's data from the past days of the current hospital stay. This type of simulated EPR allows you to examine how data for different attributes have changed over time, as well as to examine data for all of a patient's attributes at a particular time. The EPR is fully functional (as it is in a real-life hospital). You can enter such data as blood pressure, breath sounds, and certain treatments. The EPR will not, however, allow you to enter data for a previous time period. Use the arrows at the bottom of the screen to move forward and backward in time.

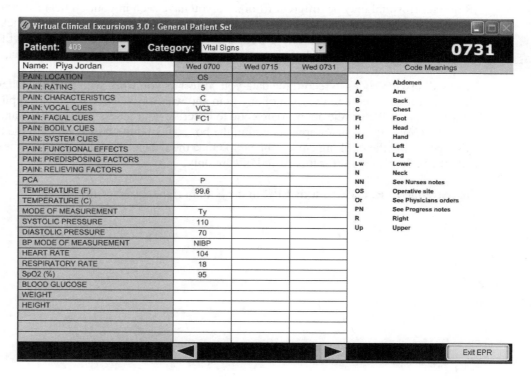

At the top of the EPR screen, you can choose patients by their room numbers. In addition, you have access to 17 different categories of patient data. To change patients or data categories, click the down arrow to the right of the room number or category.

The categories of patient data in the EPR are as follows:

- Vital Signs
- Respiratory
- Cardiovascular
- Neurologic
- Gastrointestinal
- Excretory
- Musculoskeletal
- Integumentary
- Reproductive
- Psychosocial
- Wounds and Drains
- Activity
- Hygiene and Comfort
- Safety
- Nutrition
- IV
- Intake and Output

Remember, each hospital selects its own codes. The codes used in the EPR at Pacific View Regional Hospital may be different from ones you have seen in your clinical rotations. Take some time to acquaint yourself with the codes. Within the Vital Signs category, click on any item in the left column (e.g., Pain: Characteristics). In the far-right column, you will see a list of code meanings for the possible findings and/or descriptors for that assessment area.

You will use the codes to record the data you collect as you work with patients. Click on the box in the last time column to the right of any item and wait for the code meanings applicable to that entry to appear. Select the appropriate code to describe your assessment findings and type it in the box. (*Note:* If no cursor appears within the box, click on the box again until the blue shading disappears and the blinking cursor appears.) Once the data are typed in this box, they are entered into the patient's record for this period of care only.

To leave the EPR, click on **Exit EPR** in the bottom right corner of the screen.

■ VISITING A PATIENT

From the Nurses' Station, click on the room number of the patient you wish to visit (in the tool bar at the bottom of your screen). Once you are inside the room, you will see a still photo of your patient in the top left corner. To verify that this is the correct patient, click on the **Check Armband** icon to the right of the photo. The patient's identification data will appear. If you click on **Check Allergies** (the next icon to the right), a list of the patient's allergies (if any) will replace the photo.

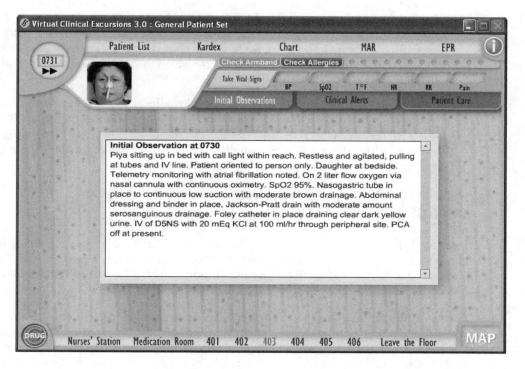

Also located in the patient's room are multiple icons you can use to assess the patient or the patient's medications. A virtual clock is provided in the upper left corner of the room to monitor your progress in real time. (*Note:* The fast-forward icon within the virtual clock will advance the time by 2-minute intervals when clicked.)

- The tool bar across the top of the screen allows you to check the **Patient List**, access the **EPR** to check or enter data, and view the patient's **Chart**, **MAR**, or **Kardex**.

- The **Take Vital Signs** icon allows you to measure the patient's up-to-the-minute blood pressure, oxygen saturation, temperature, heart rate, respiratory rate, and pain level.

- Each time you enter a patient's room, you are given an Initial Observation report to review (in the text box under the patient's photo). These notes are provided to give you a "look" at the patient as if you had just stepped into the room. You can also click on the **Initial Observations** icon to return to this box from other views within the patient's room. To the right of this icon is **Clinical Alerts**, a resource that allows you to make decisions about priority medication interventions based on emerging data collected in real time. Check this screen throughout your period of care to avoid missing critical information related to recently ordered or STAT medications.

- Clicking on **Patient Care** opens up three specific learning environments within the patient room: **Physical Assessment**, **Nurse-Client Interactions**, and **Medication Administration**.

- To perform a **Physical Assessment**, choose a body area (such as **Head & Neck**) from the column of yellow buttons. This activates a list of system subcategories for that body area (e.g., see **Sensory**, **Neurologic**, etc. in the green boxes). After you select the system you wish to evaluate, a brief description of the assessment findings will appear in a box to the right. A still photo provides a "snapshot" of how an assessment of this area might be done or what the finding might look like. For every body area, you can also click on **Equipment** on the right side of the screen.

- To the right of the Physical Assessment icon is **Nurse-Client Interactions**. Clicking on this icon will reveal the times and titles of any videos available for viewing. (*Note:* If the video you wish to see is not listed, this means you have not yet reached the correct virtual time to view that video. Check the virtual clock; you may return to access the video once its designated time has occurred—as long as you do so within the same period of care. Or you can click on the fast-forward icon within the virtual clock to advance the time by 2-minute intervals. You will then need to click again on **Patient Care** and **Nurse-Client Interactions** to refresh the screen.) To view a listed video, click on the white arrow to the right of the video title. Use the control buttons below the video to start, stop, pause, rewind, or fast-forward the action or to mute the sound.

- **Medication Administration** is the pathway that allows you to review and administer medications to a patient after you have prepared them in the Medication Room. This process is addressed further in the *How to Prepare Medications* section below and in *Medications* in the *Detailed Tour*. For additional hands-on practice, see *Reducing Medication Errors* below the *Quick* and *Detailed Tours* in your resources.

■ HOW TO QUIT, CHANGE PATIENTS, CHANGE FLOORS, OR CHANGE PERIODS OF CARE

How to Quit: From most screens, you may click the **Leave the Floor** icon on the bottom tool bar to the right of the patient room numbers. (*Note:* From some screens, you will first need to click an **Exit** button or **Return to Nurses' Station** before clicking **Leave the Floor**.) When the Floor Menu appears, click **Exit** to leave the program.

How to Change Patients, Floors, or Periods of Care: To change patients, simply click on the new patient's room number. (You cannot receive a scorecard for a new patient, however, unless you have already selected that patient on the Patient List screen.) To change to a new period of care, to change floors, or to restart the virtual clock, click on **Leave the Floor** and then on **Restart the Program**.

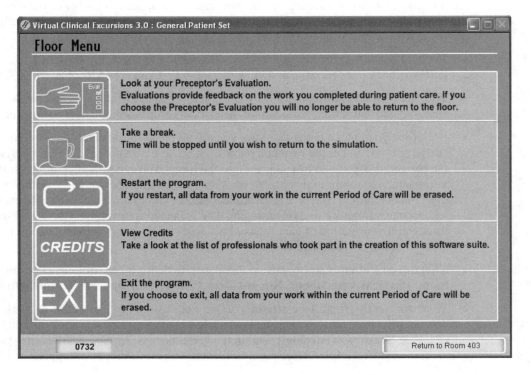

■ HOW TO PREPARE MEDICATIONS

From the Nurses' Station or the patient's room, you can access the Medication Room by clicking on the icon in the tool bar at the bottom of your screen to the left of the patient room numbers.

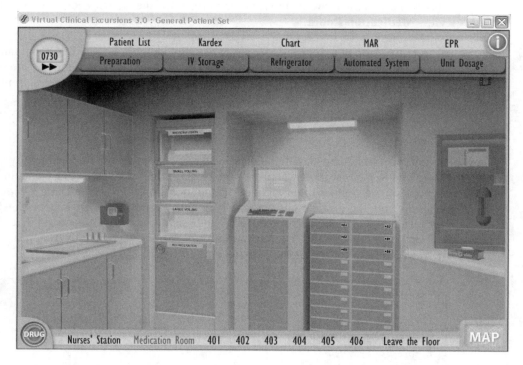

In the Medication Room you have access to the following (from left to right):

- A preparation area is located on the counter under the cabinets. To begin the medication preparation process, click on the tray on the counter or click on the **Preparation** icon at the top of the screen. The next screen leads you through a specific sequence (called the Preparation Wizard) to prepare medications one at a time for administration to a patient. However, no medication has been selected at this time. We will do this while working with a patient in *A Detailed Tour*. To exit this screen, click on **View Medication Room**.

- To the right of the cabinets (and above the refrigerator), IV storage bins are provided. Click on the bins themselves or on the **IV Storage** icon at the top of the screen. The bins are labeled **Microinfusion**, **Small Volume**, and **Large Volume**. Click on an individual bin to see a list of its contents. If you needed to prepare an IV medication at this time, you could click on the medication and its label would appear to the right under the patient's name. (*Note:* You can **Open** and **Close** any medication label by clicking the appropriate icon.) Next, you would click **Put Medication on Tray**. If you ever change your mind or decide that you have put the incorrect medication on the tray, you can reverse your actions by highlighting the medication on the tray and then clicking **Put Medication in Bin**. Click **Close Bin** in the right bottom corner to exit. **View Medication Room** brings you back to a full view of the entire room.

- A refrigerator is located under the IV storage bins to hold any medications that must be stored below room temperature. Click on the refrigerator door or on the **Refrigerator** icon at the top of the screen. Then click on the close-up view of the door to access the medications. When you are finished, click **Close Door** and then **View Medication Room**.

- To prepare controlled substances, click the **Automated System** icon at the top of the screen or click the computer monitor located to the right of the IV storage bins. A login screen will appear; your name and password are automatically filled in. Click **Login**. Select the patient for whom you wish to access medications; then select the correct medication drawer to open (they are stored alphabetically). Click **Open Drawer**, highlight the proper medication, and choose **Put Medication on Tray**. When you are finished, click **Close Drawer** and then **View Medication Room**.

- Next to the Automated System is a set of drawers identified by patient room number. To access these, click on the drawers or on the **Unit Dosage** icon at the top of the screen. This provides a close-up view of the drawers. To open a drawer, click on the room number of the patient you are working with. Next, click on the medication you would like to prepare for the patient, and a label will appear, listing the medication strength, units, and dosage per unit. To exit, click **Close Drawer**; then click **View Medication Room**.

At any time, you can learn about a medication you wish to prepare for a patient by clicking on the **Drug** icon in the bottom left corner of the medication room screen or by clicking the **Drug Guide** book on the counter to the right of the unit dosage drawers. The **Drug Guide** provides information about the medications commonly included in nursing drug handbooks. Nutritional supplements and maintenance intravenous fluid preparations are not included. Highlight a medication in the alphabetical list; relevant information about the drug will appear in the screen below. To exit, click **Return to Medication Room**.

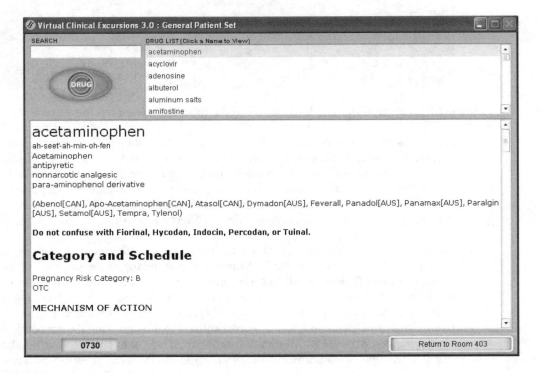

To access the MAR from the Medication Room and to review the medications ordered for a patient, click on the **MAR** icon located in the tool bar at the top of your screen and then click on the correct tab for your patient's room number. You may also click the **Review MAR** icon in the tool bar at the bottom of your screen from inside each medication storage area.

After you have chosen and prepared medications, go to the patient's room to administer them by clicking on the room number in the bottom tool bar. Inside the patient's room, click **Patient Care** and then **Medication Administration** and follow the proper administration sequence.

■ PRECEPTOR'S EVALUATIONS

When you have finished a session, click on **Leave the Floor** to go to the Floor Menu. At this point, you can click on the top icon (**Look at Your Preceptor's Evaluation**) to receive a score-card that provides feedback on the work you completed during patient care.

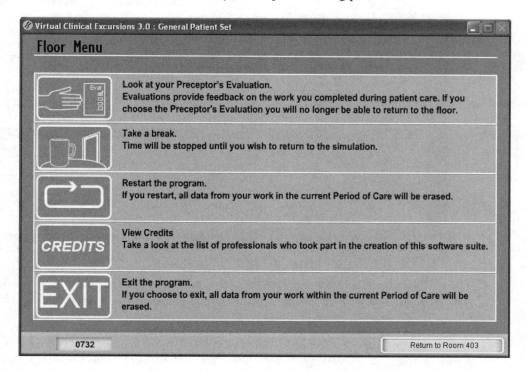

Evaluations are available for each patient you selected when you signed in for the current period of care. Click on the **Medication Scorecard** icon to see an example.

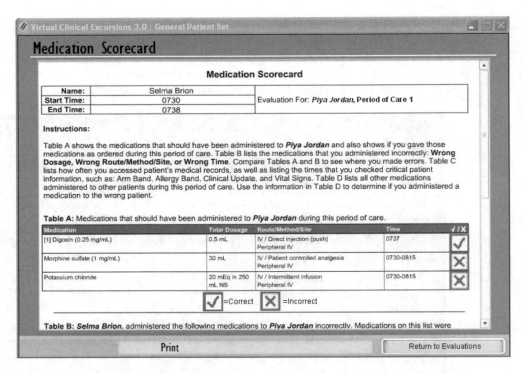

The scorecard compares the medications you administered to a patient during a period of care with what should have been administered. Table A lists the correct medications. Table B lists any medications that were administered incorrectly.

Remember, not every medication listed on the MAR should necessarily be given. For example, a patient might have an allergy to a drug that was ordered, or a medication might have been improperly transcribed to the MAR. Predetermined medication "errors" embedded within the program challenge you to exercise critical thinking skills and professional judgment when deciding to administer a medication, just as you would in a real hospital. Use all your available resources, such as the patient's chart and the MAR, to make your decision.

Table C lists the resources that were available to assist you in medication administration. It also documents whether and when you accessed these resources. For example, did you check the patient armband or perform a check of vital signs? If so, when?

You can click **Print** to get a copy of this report if needed. When you have finished reviewing the scorecard, click **Return to Evaluations** and then **Return to Menu**.

■ FLOOR MAP

To get a general sense of your location within the hospital, you can click on the **Map** icon found in the lower right corner of most of the screens in the *Virtual Clinical Excursions—General Hospital* program. (*Note:* If you are following this quick tour step by step, you will need to **Restart the Program** from the Floor Menu, sign in again, and go to the Nurses' Station to access the map.) When you click the **Map** icon, a floor map appears, showing the layout of the floor you are currently on, as well as a directory of the patients and services on that floor. As you move your cursor over the directory list, the location of each room is highlighted on the map (and vice versa). The floor map can be accessed from the Nurses' Station, Medication Room, and each patient's room.

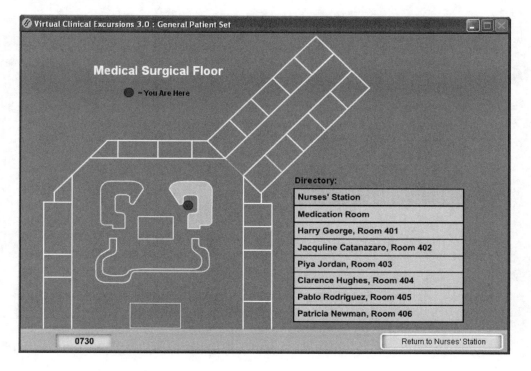

A DETAILED TOUR

If you wish to more thoroughly understand the capabilities of *Virtual Clinical Excursions—General Hospital*, take a detailed tour by completing the following section. During this tour, we will work with a specific patient to introduce you to all the different components and learning opportunities available within the software.

■ WORKING WITH A PATIENT

Sign in and select the Medical-Surgical Floor for Period of Care 1 (0730-0815). From the Patient List, select Piya Jordan and Pablo Rodriguez; however, do not go to the Nurses' Station yet.

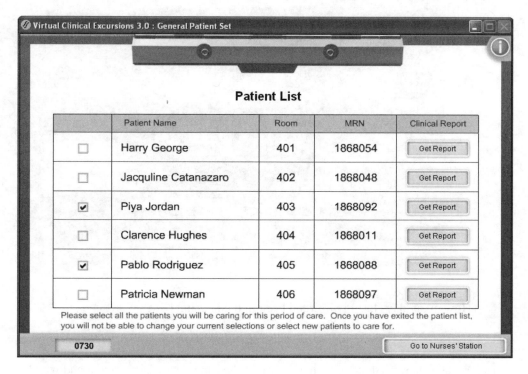

■ REPORT

In hospitals, when one shift ends and another begins, the outgoing nurse who attended a patient will give a verbal and sometimes a written summary of that patient's condition to the incoming nurse who will assume care for the patient. This summary is called a report and is an important source of data to provide an overview of a patient. Your first task is to get the clinical report on Piya Jordan. To do this, click **Get Report** in the far right column in this patient's row. From a brief review of this summary, identify the problems and areas of concern that you will need to address for this patient.

When you have finished noting any areas of concern, click on **Go to Nurses' Station**.

■ CHARTS

You can access Piya Jordan's chart from the Nurses' Station or from the patient's room (403). From the Nurses' Station, click on the chart rack or on the **Chart** icon in the tool bar at the top of your screen. Next, click on the chart labeled **403** to open the medical record for Piya Jordan. Click on the **Emergency Department** tab to view a record of why this patient was admitted.

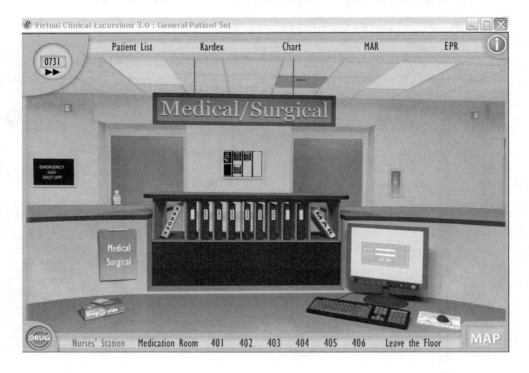

How many days has Piya Jordan been in the hospital?

What tests were done upon her arrival in the Emergency Department and why?

What was her reason for admission?

You should also click on **Diagnostic Reports** to learn what additional tests or procedures were performed and when. Finally, review the **Nursing Admission** and **History and Physical** to learn about the health history of this patient. When you are done reviewing the chart, click **Return to Nurses' Station**.

■ MEDICATIONS

Open the Medication Administration Record (MAR) by clicking on the **MAR** icon in the tool bar at the top of your screen. *Remember:* The MAR automatically opens to the first occupied room number on the floor—which is not necessarily your patient's room number! Since you need to access Piya Jordan's MAR, click on tab **403** (her room number). Always make sure you are giving the *Right Drug to the Right Patient!*

Examine the list of medications ordered for Piya Jordan. In the table below, list the medications that need to be given during this period of care (0730-0815). For each medication, note the dosage, route, and time to be given.

Time	Medication	Dosage	Route

Click on **Return to Nurses' Station**. Next, click on **403** on the bottom tool bar and then verify that you are indeed in Piya Jordan's room. Select **Clinical Alerts** (the icon to the right of Initial Observations) to check for any emerging data that might affect your medication administration priorities. Next, go to the patient's chart (click on the **Chart** icon; then click on **403**). When the chart opens, select the **Physician's Orders** tab.

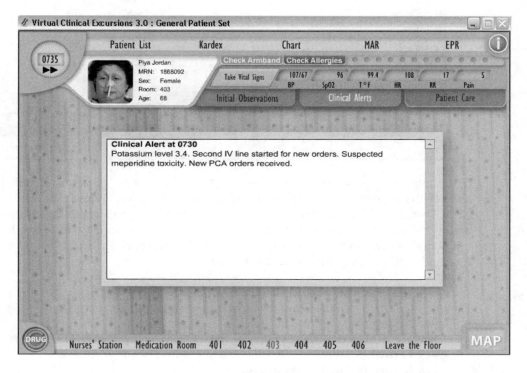

Review the orders. Have any new medications been ordered? Return to the MAR (click **Return to Room 403**; then click **MAR**). Verify that any new medications have been correctly transcribed to the MAR. Mistakes are sometimes made in the transcription process in the hospital setting, and it is sound practice to double-check any new order.

Are there any patient assessments you will need to perform before administering these medications? If so, return to Room 403 and click on **Patient Care** and then **Physical Assessment** to complete those assessments before proceeding.

Now click on the **Medication Room** icon in the tool bar at the bottom of your screen to locate and prepare the medications for Piya Jordan.

In the Medication Room, you must access the medications for Piya Jordan from the specific dispensing system in which each medication is stored. Locate each medication that needs to be given in this time period and click on **Put Medication on Tray** as appropriate. (*Hint:* Look in **Unit Dosage** drawer first.) When you are finished, click on **Close Drawer** and then on **View Medication Room**. Now click on the medication tray on the counter on the left side of the medication room screen to begin preparing the medications you have selected. (*Remember:* You can also click **Preparation** in the tool bar at the top of the screen.)

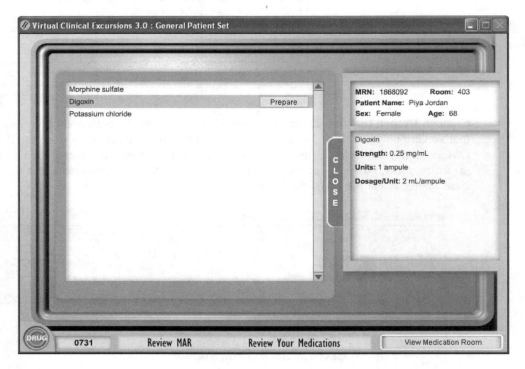

In the preparation area, you should see a list of the medications you put on the tray in the previous steps. Click on the first medication and then click **Prepare**. Follow the onscreen instructions of the Preparation Wizard, providing any data requested. As an example, let's follow the preparation process for digoxin, one of the medications due to be administered to Piya Jordan during this period of care. To begin, click to select **Digoxin**; then click **Prepare**. Now work through the Preparation Wizard sequence as detailed below:

> Amount of medication in the ampule: 2 mL.
> Enter the amount of medication you will draw up into a syringe: **0.5** mL.
> Click **Next**.
> Select the patient you wish to set aside the medication for: **Room 403, Piya Jordan**.
> Click **Finish**.
> Click **Return to Medication Room**.

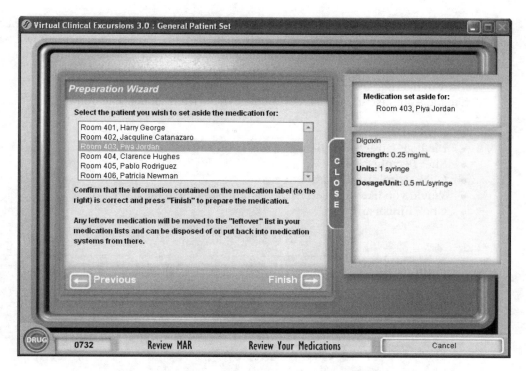

Follow this same basic process for the other medications due to be administered to Piya Jordan during this period of care. (*Hint:* Look in **IV Storage** and **Automated System**.)

PREPARATION WIZARD EXCEPTIONS

- Some medications in *Virtual Clinical Excursions—General Hospital* are prepared by the pharmacy (e.g., IV antibiotics) and taken to the patient room as a whole. This is common practice in most hospitals.
- Blood products are not administered by students through the *Virtual Clinical Excursions—General Hospital* simulations since blood administration follows specific protocols not covered in this program.
- The *Virtual Clinical Excursions—General Hospital* simulations do not allow for mixing more than one type of medication, such as regular and Lente insulins, in the same syringe. In the clinical setting, when multiple types of insulin are ordered for a patient, the regular insulin is drawn up first, followed by the longer-acting insulin. Insulin is always administered in a special unit-marked syringe.

Now return to Room 403 (click on **403** on the bottom tool bar) to administer Piya Jordan's medications.

At any time during the medication administration process, you can perform a further review of systems, take vital signs, check information contained within the chart, or verify patient identity and allergies. Inside Piya Jordan's room, click **Take Vital Signs**. (*Note:* These findings change over time to reflect the temporal changes you would find in a patient similar to Piya Jordan.)

When you have gathered all the data you need, click on **Patient Care** and then select **Medication Administration**. Any medications you prepared in the previous steps should be listed on the left side of your screen. Let's continue the administration process with the digoxin ordered for Piya Jordan. Click to highlight **Digoxin** in the list of medications. Next, click on the down arrow to the right of **Select** and choose **Administer** from the drop-down menu. This will activate the Administration Wizard. Complete the Wizard sequence as follows:

- Route: **IV**
- Method: **Direct Injection**
- Site: **Peripheral IV**
- Click **Administer to Patient** arrow.
- Would you like to document this administration in the MAR? **Yes**
- Click **Finish** arrow.

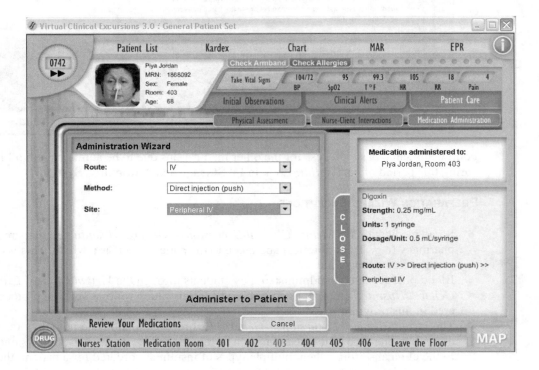

Your selections are recorded by a tracking system and evaluated on a Medication Scorecard stored under Preceptor's Evaluations. This scorecard can be viewed, printed, and given to your instructor. To access the Preceptor's Evaluations, click on **Leave the Floor**. When the Floor Menu appears, select **Look at Your Preceptor's Evaluation**. Then click on **Medication Scorecard** inside the box with Piya Jordan's name (see example on the following page).

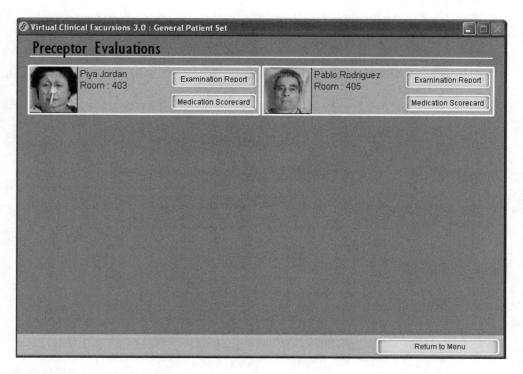

■ MEDICATION SCORECARD

- First, review Table A. Was digoxin given correctly? Did you give the other medications as ordered?
- Table B shows you which (if any) medications you gave incorrectly.
- Table C addresses the resources used for Piya Jordan. Did you access the patient's chart, MAR, EPR, or Kardex as needed to make safe medication administration decisions?
- Did you check the patient's armband to verify her identity? Did you check whether your patient had any known allergies to medications? Were vital signs taken?

When you have finished reviewing the scorecard, click **Return to Evaluations** and then **Return to Menu**.

■ VITAL SIGNS

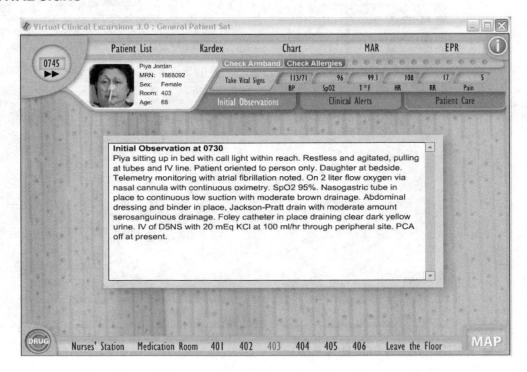

Vital signs, often considered the traditional "signs of life," include body temperature, heart rate, respiratory rate, blood pressure, oxygen saturation of the blood, and pain level.

Inside Piya Jordan's room, click **Take Vital Signs**. (*Note:* If you are following this detailed tour step by step, you will need to **Restart the Program** from the Floor Menu, sign in again for Period of Care 1, and navigate to Room 403.) Collect vital signs for this patient and record them below. Note the time at which you collected each of these data. (*Remember:* You can take vital signs at any time. The data change over time to reflect the temporal changes you would find in a patient similar to Piya Jordan.)

Vital Signs	Findings/Time
Blood pressure	
O$_2$ saturation	
Temperature	
Heart rate	
Respiratory rate	
Pain rating	

After you are done, click on the **EPR** icon located in the tool bar at the top of the screen. Your username and password are automatically provided. Click on **Login** to enter the EPR. To access Piya Jordan's records, click on the down arrow next to Patient and choose her room number, **403**. Select **Vital Signs** as the category. Next, in the empty time column on the far right, record the vital signs data you just collected in Piya Jordan's room. If you need help with this process, refer to the Electronic Patient Record (EPR) section of the Quick Tour. Now compare these findings with the data you collected earlier for this patient's vital signs. Use these earlier findings to establish a baseline for each of the vital signs.

    a.   Are any of the data you collected significantly different from the baseline for a particular vital sign?

         Circle One: Yes   No

    b.   If "Yes," which data are different?

■ PHYSICAL ASSESSMENT

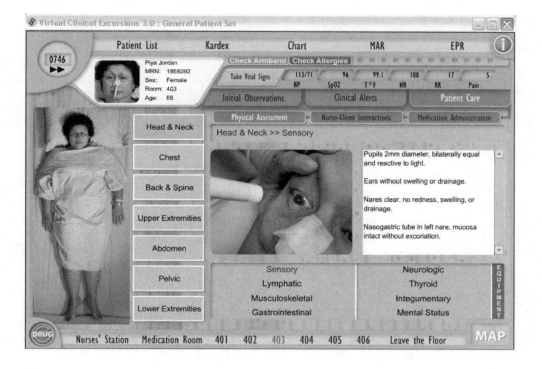

After you have finished examining the EPR for vital signs, click **Exit EPR** to return to Room 403. Click **Patient Care** and then **Physical Assessment**. Think about the information you received in the report at the beginning of this shift, as well as what you may have learned about this patient from the chart. Based on this, what area(s) of examination should you pay most attention to at this time? Is there any equipment you should be monitoring? Conduct a physical assessment of the body areas and systems that you consider priorities for Piya Jordan. For example, select **Head & Neck**; then click on and assess **Sensory** and **Lymphatic**. Complete any other assessment(s) you think are necessary at this time. In the following table, record the data you collected during this examination.

Area of Examination	Findings
Head & Neck Sensory	
Head & Neck Lymphatic	

After you have finished collecting these data, return to the EPR. Compare the data that were already in the record with those you just collected.

   a. Are any of the data you collected significantly different from the baselines for this patient?

      Circle One: Yes   No

   b. If "Yes," which data are different?

■ NURSE-CLIENT INTERACTIONS

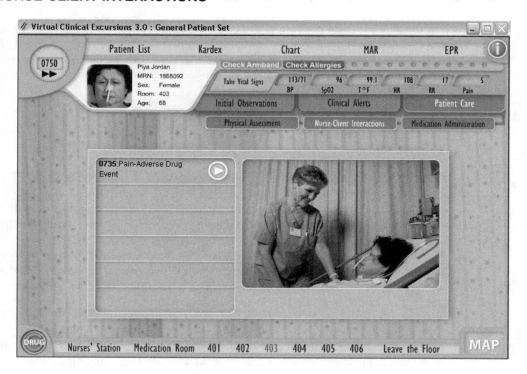

Click on **Patient Care** from inside Piya Jordan's room (403). Now click on **Nurse-Client Interactions** to access a short video titled **Pain—Adverse Drug Event**, which is available for viewing at or after 0735 (based on the virtual clock in the upper left corner of your screen; see *Note* below.). To begin the video, click on the white arrow next to its title. You will observe a nurse communicating with Piya Jordan and her daughter. There are many variations of nursing practice, some exemplifying "best" practice and some not. Note whether the nurse in this inter-action displays professional behavior and compassionate care. Are her words congruent with what is going on with the patient? Does this interaction "feel right" to you? If not, how would you handle this situation differently? Explain.

Note: If the video you wish to view is not listed, this means you have not yet reached the correct virtual time to view that video. Check the virtual clock; you may return to access the video once its designated time has occurred—as long as you do so within the same period of care. Or you can click on the fast-forward icon within the virtual clock to advance the time by 2-minute inter-vals. You will then need to click again on **Patient Care** and **Nurse-Client Interactions** to refresh the screen.

At least one Nurse-Client Interactions video is available during each period of care. Viewing these videos can help you learn more about what is occurring with a patient at a certain time and also prompt you to discern between nurse communications that are ideal and those that need improvement. Compassionate care and the ability to communicate clearly are essential compo-nents of delivering quality nursing care, and it is during your clinical time that you will begin to refine these skills.

■ COLLECTING AND EVALUATING DATA

Each of the activities you perform in the Patient Care environment generates a significant amount of assessment data. Remember that after you collect data, you can record your findings in the EPR. You can also review the EPR, patient's chart, videos, and MAR at any time. You will get plenty of practice collecting and then evaluating data in context of the patient's course.

Now, here's an important question for you:

> Did the previous sequence of exercises provide the most efficient way to assess Piya Jordan?

For example, you went to the patient's room to get vital signs, then back to the EPR to enter data and compare your findings with extant data. Next, you went back to the patient's room to do a physical examination, then again back to the EPR to enter and review data. If this back-and-forth process of data collection and recording seemed inefficient, remember the following:

- Plan all of your nursing activities to maximize efficiency, while at the same time optimizing the quality of patient care. (Think about what data you might need before performing certain tasks. For example, do you need to check a heart rate before administering a cardiac medication or check an IV site before starting an infusion?)

- You collect a tremendous amount of data when you work with a patient. Very few people can accurately remember all these data for more than a few minutes. Develop efficient assessment skills, and record data as soon as possible after collecting them.

- Assessment data are only the starting point for the nursing process.

Make a clear distinction between these first exercises and how you actually provide nursing care. These initial exercises were designed to involve you actively in the use of different software components. This workbook focuses on sensible practices for implementing the nursing process in ways that ensure the highest-quality care of patients.

Most important, remember that a human being changes through time, and that these changes include both the physical and psychosocial facets of a person as a living organism. Think about this for a moment. Some patients may change physically in a very short time (a patient with emerging myocardial infarction) or more slowly (a patient with a chronic illness). Patients' overall physical and psychosocial conditions may improve or deteriorate. They may have effective coping skills and familial support, or they may feel alone and full of despair. In fact, each individual is a complex mix of physical and psychosocial elements, and at least some of these elements usually change through time.

Thus it is crucial that you *DO NOT* think of the nursing process as a simple one-time, five-step procedure consisting of assessment, nursing diagnosis, planning, implementation, and evaluation. Rather, the nursing process should be utilized as a creative and systematic approach to delivering nursing care. Furthermore, because all living organisms are constantly changing, we must apply the nursing process over and over. Each time we follow the nursing process for an individual patient, we refine our understanding of that patient's physical and psychosocial conditions based on collection and analysis of many different types of data. *Virtual Clinical Excursions—General Hospital* will help you develop both the creativity and the systematic approach needed to become a nurse who is equipped to deliver the highest-quality care to all patients.

REDUCING MEDICATION ERRORS

Earlier in the detailed tour, you learned the basic steps of medication preparation and administration. The following simulations will allow you to practice those skills further—with an increased emphasis on reducing medication errors by using the Medication Scorecard to evaluate your work.

Sign in to work on the Medical-Surgical Floor at Pacific View Regional Hospital for Period of Care 1. (*Note:* If you are already working with another patient or during another period of care, click on **Leave the Floor** and then **Restart the Program**; then sign in.)

From the Patient List, select Clarence Hughes. Then click on **Go to Nurses' Station**. Complete the following steps to prepare and administer medications to Clarence Hughes.

- Click on **Medication Room** on the tool bar at the bottom of your screen.
- Click on **MAR** and then on tab **404** to determine medications that have been ordered for Clarence Hughes. (*Note:* You may click on **Review MAR** at any time to verify the correct medication order. Always remember to check the patient name on the MAR to make sure you have the correct patient's record. You must click on the correct room number tab within the MAR.) Click on **Return to Medication Room** after reviewing the correct MAR.
- Click on **Unit Dosage** (or on the Unit Dosage cabinet); from the close-up view, click on drawer **404**.
- Select the medications you would like to administer. After each selection, click **Put Medication on Tray**. When you are finished selecting medications, click **Close Drawer** and then **View Medication Room**.
- Click on **Automated System** (or on the Automated System unit itself). Click **Login**.
- On the next screen, specify the correct patient and drawer location.
- Select the medication you would like to administer and click on **Put Medication on Tray**. Repeat this process if you wish to administer other medications from the Automated System.
- When you are finished, click **Close Drawer** and **View Medication Room**.
- From the Medication Room, click on **Preparation** (or on the preparation tray).
- From the list of medications on your tray, highlight the correct medication to administer and click **Prepare**.
- This activates the Preparation Wizard. Supply any requested information; then click **Next**.
- Now select the correct patient to receive this medication and click **Finish**.
- Repeat the previous three steps until all medications that you want to administer are prepared.
- You can click on **Review Your Medications** and then on **Return to Medication Room** when ready. Once you are back in the Medication Room, go directly to Clarence Hughes' room by clicking on **404** at bottom of screen.
- Inside the patient's room, administer the medication, utilizing the six rights of medication administration. After you have collected the appropriate assessment data and are ready for administration, click **Patient Care** and then **Medication Administration**. Verify that the correct patient and medication(s) appear in the left-hand window. Highlight the first medication you wish to administer; then click the down arrow next to Select. From the drop-down menu, select **Administer** and complete the Administration Wizard by providing any information requested. When the Wizard stops asking for information, click **Administer to Patient**. Specify **Yes** when asked whether this administration should be recorded in the MAR. Finally, click **Finish**.

■ **SELF-EVALUATION**

Now let's see how you did during your medication administration!

- Click on **Leave the Floor** at the bottom of your screen. From the Floor Menu, select **Look at Your Preceptor's Evaluation**. Then click **Medication Scorecard**.

The following exercises will help you identify medication errors, investigate possible reasons for these errors, and reduce or prevent medication errors in the future.

1. Start by examining Table A. These are the medications you should have given to Clarence Hughes during this period of care. If each of the medications in Table A has a ✓ by it, then you made no errors. Congratulations!

If any medication has an X by it, then you made one or more medication errors.

Compare Tables A and B to determine which of the following types of errors you made: Wrong Dose, Wrong Route/Method/Site, or Wrong Time. Follow these steps:
   a. Find medications in Table A that were given incorrectly.
   b. Now see if those same medications are in Table B, which shows what you actually administered to Clarence Hughes.
   c. Comparing Tables A and B, match the Strength, Dose, Route/Method/Site, and Time for each medication you administered incorrectly.
   d. Then, using the form below, list the medications given incorrectly and mark the errors you made for each medication.

Medication	Strength	Dosage	Route	Method	Site	Time
	❑	❑	❑	❑	❑	❑
	❑	❑	❑	❑	❑	❑
	❑	❑	❑	❑	❑	❑
	❑	❑	❑	❑	❑	❑

2. To help you reduce future medication errors, consider the following list of possible reasons for errors.

- Did not check drug against MAR for correct medication, correct dose, correct patient, correct route, correct time, correct documentation.
- Did not check drug dose against MAR three times.
- Did not open the unit dose package in the patient's room.
- Did not correctly identify the patient using two identifiers.
- Did not administer the drug on time.
- Did not verify patient allergies.
- Did not check the patient's current condition or vital sign parameters.
- Did not consider why the patient would be receiving this drug.
- Did not question why the drug was in the patient's drawer.
- Did not check the physician's order and/or check with the pharmacist when there was a question about the drug or dose.
- Did not verify that no adverse effects had occurred from a previous dose.

Based on the list of possibilities you just reviewed, determine how you made each error and record the reason in the form below:

Medication	Reason for Error

3. Look again at Table B. Are there medications listed that are not in Table A? If so, you gave a medication to Clarence Hughes that he should not have received. Complete the following exercises to help you understand how such an error might have been made.

   a. Perhaps you gave a medication that was on Clarence Hughes' MAR for this period of care, without recognizing that a change had occurred in the patient's condition, which should have caused you to reconsider. Review patient records as necessary and complete the following form:

Medication	Possible Reasons Not to Give This Medication

   b. Another possibility is that you gave Clarence Hughes a medication that should have been given at a different time. Check his MAR and complete the form below to determine whether you made a Wrong Time error:

Medication	Given to Clarence Hughes at What Time	Should Have Been Given at What Time

c. Maybe you gave another patient's medication to Clarence Hughes. In this case, you made a Wrong Patient error. Check the MARs of other patients and use the form below to determine whether you made this type of error:

Medication	Given to Clarence Hughes	Should Have Been Given to

4. The Medication Scorecard provides some other interesting sources of information. For example, if there is a medication selected for Clarence Hughes but it was not given to him, there will be an X by that medication in Table A, but it will not appear in Table B. In that case, you might have given this medication to some other patient, which is another type of Wrong Patient error. To investigate further, look at Table D, which lists the medications you gave to other patients. See whether you can find any medications ordered for Clarence Hughes that were given to another patient by mistake. However, before you make any decisions, be sure to cross-check the MAR for other patients because the same medication may have been ordered for multiple patients. Use the following form to record your findings:

Medication	Should Have Been Given to Clarence Hughes	Given by Mistake to

5. Now take some time to review the medication exercises you just completed. Use the form below to create an overall analysis of what you have learned. Once again, record each of the medication errors you made, including the type of each error. Then, for each error you made, indicate specifically what you would do differently to prevent this type of error from occurring again.

Medication	Type of Error	Error Prevention Tactic

Submit this form to your instructor if required as a graded assignment, or simply use these exercises to improve your understanding of medication errors and how to reduce them.

Name: _____   Date: _____

KEY ICONS

The following icons are used throughout this workbook to help you quickly identify particular activities and assignments:

 Indicates a reading assignment—tells you which textbook chapter(s) you should read before starting each lesson

 Indicates a writing activity

 Marks the beginning of an interactive virtual hospital activity—signals you to return to your *Virtual Clinical Excursions* simulation

 Indicates additional virtual hospital activity instructions

 Indicates questions and activities that require you to consult your textbook

 Indicates the approximate time required to complete an exercise

LESSON 1 —————————————

Caring Throughout the Lifespan

_____

 Reading Assignment: Developmental Theories (Chapter 11)
Young and Middle Adults (Chapter 13)
Older Adult (Chapter 14)
Patient Safety (Chapter 27)

Patients: Clarence Hughes, Medical-Surgical Floor, Room 404
William Jefferson, Skilled Nursing Floor, Room 501

Objectives:

1. Describe physiologic changes of aging.
2. Identify developmental tasks of adults.
3. Differentiate between dementia, delirium, and depression.
4. Discuss older adult health concerns as they apply to two patients.
5. Discuss safety risks as they apply to two patients.
6. Develop a plan of care for an older adult with safety risks.

Exercise 1

Writing Activity

15 minutes

1. Identify the stages of adulthood. Include the age range for each stage.

2. A student nurse is preparing a presentation concerning the "sandwich generation." Which of the following statements about this concept is correct?
   a. The name is derived from the amount of fast food consumed by this generation.
   b. Members of the sandwich generation include school-age children.
   c. Adults in their middle years are members of this category.
   d. Elder adults are members of the sandwich generation.

3. _____ Intellectual decline is a normal part of aging. (True/False)

4. The leading cause of death for older adults is:
   a. heart disease.
   b. unintentional injuries.
   c. acquired immunodeficiency syndrome (AIDS).
   d. bone cancer.

5. A middle-aged female patient asks about her risk for osteoporosis during this period in her life. Which of the following is the best response by the nurse?
   a. "Osteoporosis is not a concern until late adulthood."
   b. "Osteoporosis is only an issue for underweight women."
   c. "Osteoporosis is a greater concern for young women of childbearing age."
   d. "It is too late to prevent osteoporosis-related complications."
   e. "Osteoporosis is a concern for women of this age."

Exercise 2

Virtual Hospital Activity

45 minutes

- Sign in to work at Pacific View Regional Hospital on the Skilled Nursing Floor for Period of Care 1. (*Note:* If you are already in the virtual hospital from a previous exercise, click on **Leave the Floor** and then on **Restart the Program** to get to the sign-in window.)
- From the Patient List, select William Jefferson (Room 501).
- Click on **Get Report**; review the report and then click on **Go to Nurses' Station**.
- Click on **Chart** and then on **501**.
- Click on and then review the **Nursing Admission** and the **History & Physical**.

1. Who is William Jefferson? Why has he been admitted to the Skilled Nursing Unit?

2. List four developmental tasks that pose difficulties for William Jefferson. State your rationale for choosing each task.

3. William Jefferson takes eight different medications ordered by his physician. Polypharmacy increases his risk for adverse drug reactions. Explain what you would do to ensure that he takes his medications safely and appropriately once he returns home.

4. William Jefferson has a hearing loss in his left ear. Which of the following actions will promote positive communication? Select all that apply.

   _____ Always speak toward the ear affected by the hearing loss.

   _____ Check the ear for cerumen impaction.

   _____ Speak in a clear, high-pitched tone at a higher volume.

   _____ Reduce background noise during a discussion.

   _____ Encourage patient to wear his hearing devices during a conversation.

5. The record indicates that William Jefferson has experienced delirium.

   a. What was the most likely cause of his delirium?

b. What other factors might have contributed to the delirium?

c. How does delirium differ from dementia in regard to the following: onset, progression, orientation, and memory?

d. Patients with Alzheimer's disease frequently also suffer from depression. Depression can be distinguished from both dementia and delirium in what ways?

6. Nursing assessment of a patient with dementia and delirium is especially complex when an aging patient also suffers from chronic disease. Critical thinking applied to assessment enables a nurse to identify relevant nursing diagnoses. Complete the following critical thinking diagram for assessment of William Jefferson by writing the letter of each critical thinking factor on one of the lines under its proper category.

Knowledge

1. _____

2. _____

3. _____

Experience

Assessment of William Jefferson

Standards

4. _____

5. _____

6. _____

Attitudes

7. _____

8. _____

Critical Thinking Factors

a. Ask the patient's wife to describe how his sleep is affected when he becomes anxious or fearful.

b. Consider the effects diabetes has on physical assessment findings for vascular and neurologic function.

c. Reflect on previous encounters when you have assessed confused patients.

d. Introduce yourself when you begin to assess William Jefferson and use a calm, steady approach, explaining each step with conviction.

e. Refer to a gerontology textbook for the characteristics of dementia.

f. Take time in assessing William Jefferson, do not rush, and examine all body systems thoroughly.

g. Consider the effects William Jefferson's medications have on physical findings.

h. When assessing the patient's level of discomfort, always use a pain scale.

➡ • Click on **Return to Nurses' Station**.

• Select Room **501** at the bottom of the screen.

• Review the Initial Observations.

• Click on **Patient Care** and then on **Nurse-Client Interactions**.

• Select and view the video titled **0730: Intervention—Patient Safety**. (*Note:* Check the virtual clock to see whether enough time has elapsed. You can use the fast-forward feature to advance the time by 2-minute intervals if the video is not yet available. Then click again on **Patient Care** and on **Nurse-Client Interactions** to refresh the screen.)

7. Which of the following fall risks apply to William Jefferson? Select all that apply.

_____ History of falls

_____ Confusion

_____ Age (over 65)

_____ Impaired judgment

_____ Sensory deficit

_____ Unable to ambulate independently

_____ Decreased level of cooperation

_____ Increased anxiety

_____ Incontinence

_____ Medications affecting blood pressure or consciousness

_____ Postural hypotension with dizziness

8. Based on what you know about William Jefferson's condition, complete the following care plan for the nursing diagnosis Risk for Falls. Provide a goal, two expected outcomes, and three interventions relevant to this patient's situation.

Nursing Diagnosis: Risk for Falls

Goal

Expected Outcomes

1.

2.

Interventions

1.

2.

3.

9. Which of the following devices would be useful in protecting William Jefferson from falling as he gets out of bed?
   a. Vail-enclosed bed
   b. Jacket restraint
   c. Ambularm
   d. Full set of side rails

 10. Determine William Jefferson's fall risk score. Explain your scoring. (*Hint:* See Table 27-1 in your textbook.)

Exercise 3

 Virtual Hospital Activity

 30 minutes

- Sign in to work at Pacific View Regional Hospital on the Medical-Surgical Floor for Period of Care 1. (*Note:* If you are already in the virtual hospital from a previous exercise, click on **Leave the Floor** and then on **Restart the Program** to get to the sign-in window.)
- From the Patient List, select Clarence Hughes (Room 404).
- Click on **Get Report**; review the report and then click on **Go to Nurses' Station**.
- Click on **Chart** and then on **404**.
- Click on and then review the **History and Physical**.

1. Who is Clarence Hughes and why has he been admitted to the hospital?

 - Click on **Nurse's Notes**. Review the note for Wednesday at 0715.

2. Clarence Hughes has reported feeling constipated. What normal physiologic change of aging might contribute to this problem? How might Clarence Hughes' osteoarthritis further contribute to constipation?

3. Clarence Hughes has a history of smoking, which adds to his risk for respiratory problems. Which of the following respiratory changes are considered normal physiologic changes associated with aging? Select all that apply. (*Hint:* See Table 14-1 in your textbook.)

_____ Increased number of alveoli

_____ Decreased cough reflex

_____ Decreased vital capacity

_____ Increased removal of mucus

_____ Increased airway resistance

_____ Increased risk for respiratory infections

→ • Click on and then review the **Nursing Admission**.

4. Chronic disease diminishes the well-being of older adults. Identify three nursing interventions focusing on prevention that would be appropriate for Clarence Hughes.

5. After reviewing Clarence Hughes' admission data, describe how he has been able to meet each of the following developmental tasks.

Maintaining quality of life

Redefining relationships with adult children

LESSON 2
_____

Critical Thinking in Nursing Practice

 Reading Assignment: Critical Thinking in Nursing Practice (Chapter 15)
Nursing Assessment (Chapter 16)

Patient: Harry George, Medical-Surgical Floor, Room 401

Objectives:

1. Describe characteristics of a critical thinker.
2. Discuss the nurse's responsibility in making clinical decisions.
3. Discuss the critical thinking skills used in nursing practice.
4. Discuss the relationship of the nursing process to critical thinking.
5. Differentiate between subjective and objective data.
6. Review the use of interview techniques when collecting data from a patient.
7. Describe the components of a nursing history.

Exercise 1

Writing Activity

30 minutes

1. _____ is based on research or clinical
   experience.

2. The purpose of the assessment is to establish a(n) _____ about a patient's
   perceived needs, health problems, and responses to these problems.

3. When providing care to a patient, a nurse should attempt to assess for the presence of
   relationships between findings. This practice is known as:
   a. interpretation.
   b. analysis.
   c. inference.
   d. evaluation.

4. Name at least five characteristics a nurse must employ when acting as a critical thinker.

5. A graduate nurse has begun to demonstrate the characteristics of a complex critical thinker. Based on your knowledge of this process, what characteristics will the nurse likely demonstrate?
   a. An expectation that an expert will have a correct answer for problems encountered
   b. An ability and desire to follow procedures in a step-by-step manner
   c. The ability to review the implications of each potential intervention
   d. The realization of the need to make decisions without help from others

6. The graduate nurse notices that his preceptor regularly seeks additional information from peers to make a decision. Which critical thinking activity is being demonstrated by the preceptor?
   a. Humility
   b. Confidence
   c. Perseverance
   d. Curiosity
   e. Integrity

7. The nurse is completing the initial assessment for a patient recently admitted to the inpatient unit. Which of the following best expresses the rationale for this activity?
   a. To determine the patient's goals
   b. To identify the patient's problems
   c. To evaluate the patient's condition
   d. To set desired outcomes for the patient for the care being delivered

8. In caring for the patient, nonverbal behaviors can be a valuable additive to the nurse-patient relationship. Can you identify these behaviors?

9. _____ refers to the process of comparing data with other sources to determine accuracy.

10. The nurse is reviewing data collected from the patient during the admission process. Which of the following findings will be included in the environmental history? Select all that apply.

_____ Available resources to be used after discharge

_____ Religious practices

_____ Family structure within the home

_____ Lifestyle patterns

_____ History of tobacco use

_____ Placement of bath facilities within the home

_____ Exposure to heavy metals in the workplace

11. _____ Back channeling is a technique that patients will often view as rude or inattentive. (True/False)

12. _____ A patient of Middle Eastern descent who possesses traditional values may find it rude if the nurse does not maintain firm eye contact. (True/False)

13. _____ The reason for seeking medical care and the patient's expectations for the care are not necessarily the same. (True/False)

14. Match each phase of the nursing process with the appropriate description.

Nursing Process	Description
_____ Assessment	a. Set goals of care and desired outcomes.
_____ Diagnosis	b. Identify the patient's problems.
_____ Plan	c. Gather information about the patient's condition.
_____ Implementation	d. Determine whether goals are met and have been achieved.
_____ Evaluation	e. Perform the nursing actions identified in planning.

15. After completing the data collection, the nurse is preparing to analyze the data. What steps should be included in the analysis of the data?

Exercise 2

Virtual Hospital Activity

30 minutes

- Sign in to work at Pacific View Regional Hospital on the Medical-Surgical Floor for Period of Care 1. (*Note:* If you are already in the virtual hospital from a previous exercise, click on **Leave the Floor** and then on **Restart the Program** to get to the sign-in window.)
- From the Patient List, select Harry George (Room 401).
- Click on **Get Report** and review.
- Click on **Go to Nurses' Station**.
- Click on **Chart** and select the chart for Room **401**.
- Click on and review the **Nursing Admission**.

1. What are Harry George's medical diagnoses?

2. _____ In the nursing admission and history, Harry George has reported, "My foot has been killing me, and nothing helps the pain." This is an example of an objective patient report. (True/False)

3. In addition to Harry George himself, what other sources of data may be used when gathering information to develop the plan of care?

• Still in the Nursing Admissions section of the chart, review the nurse's description of the patient's left leg wound made upon admission.

   • Next, click on **Consultations** and review the note from the wound care team.

4. Intellectual standards of critical thinking are commonly applied when assessing a patient. Compare the Nursing Admission description of Harry George's left foot in the progress note with the description in the wound care consultation. Which note was more complete? Why?

5. A review of the data indicates a discrepancy between the measurement of Harry George's wound recorded by the nurse and the wound care team. The best initial action by the nurse will be to:
   a. leave a note for the physician pointing out the differences in the measurements.
   b. notify the nursing supervisor regarding the discrepancies in the measurements.
   c. contact the wound care team to discuss the discrepancy.
   d. measure the wound to validate the nursing documentation.

6. After collecting assessment data from Harry George and validating for accuracy, you may begin to interpret the clinical information by organizing it into meaningful:
   a. inferences.
   b. problems.
   c. clusters.
   d. nursing diagnoses.

 • Click on **Return to Nurses' Station**.

   • Click on **EPR** and **Login**.

   • Select **401** from the Patient drop-down menu and **Vital Signs** from the Category drop-down menu.

   • Review the data from Monday at 1835 to Wednesday at 0700.

   • Change the Category to **Nutrition** and review the data for the same time frame.

7. Certain cues can be used to signal patterns that suggest a nursing diagnosis. After reviewing data from the nursing history and the EPR, match each defining characteristic below with the corresponding data cluster from Harry George's admission history.

Defining Characteristic	**Admission Data Cluster**
_____ Verbal report	a. Change in sleep cycle
_____ Sore inflamed buccal cavity	b. Groans
_____ Lack of interest in food	c. Eats one meal a day
_____ Expressive behavior	d. "My foot is killing me"
_____ Sleep disturbance	e. Gums dark pink, swollen
_____ Reported food intake less than RDA	f. "Haven't felt like eating for the last week"

8. In the Nursing Admission, Harry George's sleep pattern is documented as being "irregular, never more than 2 hours." You decide to question the patient further about the sleep habits he follows—for example, what time he normally goes to bed, his activities before going to sleep, the number of times he awakens during the night. Your decision is an example of what critical thinking attitude?

_____ Humility

_____ Thinking independently

_____ Risk taking

_____ Perseverance

→ • Click on **Exit EPR**.
   • Click on **Chart** and select the chart for Room **401**.
   • Click on and review the **History and Physical**.

9. Critical thinking involves applying knowledge to best analyze and understand the patient's problems. After considering the physician's medical plan, list four areas of knowledge that would help you to support the plan of care.

→ • Click on **Return to Nurses' Station**.
   • Click on **401** at the bottom of the screen.
   • Click on **Patient Care** and then on **Physical Assessment**.
   • Select **Lower Extremities** and review the assessment findings.

10. After reviewing the condition of Harry George's wound, the conclusion as to whether the wound is healing is an example of _____.

11. When you see a change in the wound from reddened margins to clear and less inflamed, you make a(n) _____ from this evidence in order to conclude the wound is healing.

12. After applying saline to Harry George's wound over 2 days, your evaluation of the use of saline over time is an example of _____.

13. If you, as the nurse, questioned the wound care team's recommendations for a dressing for Harry George, you would be demonstrating the critical thinking attitude of

_____.

14. Given Harry George's relationship with his children, what should their role be in his plan of care?

15. Consider Maslow's hierarchy when planning Harry George's plan of care. What stages of development is Harry George working on at this time?

Planning and Application of the Nursing Process

 Reading Assignment: Nursing Assessment (Chapter 16)
Nursing Diagnosis (Chapter 17)
Planning Nursing Care (Chapter 18)
Implementing Nursing Care (Chapter 19)
Evaluation (Chapter 20)
Documentation and Informatics (Chapter 26, pages 357-358)

Patient: Patricia Newman, Medical-Surgical Floor, Room 406

Objectives:

1. Assess the health care needs of two patients.
2. Develop nursing diagnoses from available data.
3. Identify priorities of nursing care for two patients.
4. Develop goals and outcome statements.
5. Discuss factors to consider in choosing nursing interventions.

Exercise 1

 Writing Activity

 30 minutes

1. A nurse is preparing to start her shift on a medical-surgical unit. Which of the following factors concerning the change-of-shift report (hand-off report) will be most important for the nurse to consider? (*Hint:* See pages 357-358 in your textbook.)
   a. Next anticipated dressing change
   b. Patient's personality
   c. Patient's family support
   d. Off-going nurse's opinion about the patient's family background

2. _____ Physiologic diagnoses have a higher priority than psychologic diagnoses. (True/False)

3. _____ The Kardex provides a filing system for recording the physician's orders. (True/False)

4. When providing care to the patient, it is important for the nurse to be able to exercise

   _____, which allow the practitioner to shift
   attention to differing concerns during a period of care.

5. The statement that outlines the desired change in the patient's condition or behavior is

   termed the _____. (*Hint:* See page 238 in your textbook.)

6. You are assigned to provide care to a patient who has recently had abdominal surgery. When
   you are updating the nursing care plan, which of the following patient outcomes would be
   appropriate to include? Select all that apply.

   _____ The nurse will observe the patient's understanding of use of the incentive
   spirometry.

   _____ The patient will demonstrate an increased level of comfort.

   _____ The patient will initiate turning and deep breathing within 2 hours.

   _____ The patient will be more comfortable.

   _____ The patient will report lessened pain using the pain scale within 3 hours.

7. A review of the care planned for a patient during a given shift reveals the interventions
   listed below. Which of these interventions is classified as an independent nursing intervention? Select all that apply.

   _____ Anchor an indwelling Foley catheter.

   _____ Discontinue IV.

   _____ Refer the patient for home health care.

   _____ Review complications to report after discharge.

   _____ Record intake and output.

8. List the seven domains that may be used to classify nursing interventions.

9. The nurse is assisting a newly graduated nurse in completing a care plan. Which of the nursing interventions planned by the graduate and listed below indicate the need for further instruction? Select all that apply.

_____ Push fluids.

_____ Monitor blood pressure.

_____ Monitor blood pressure every 4 hours.

_____ Call physician for elevated temperature.

_____ Assist patient to turn, cough, and deep-breathe every 2 hours.

10. A(n) _____ is a preprinted form with orders for routine therapies, monitoring guidelines, and/or diagnostic procedures for specific patients with identified clinical problems.

11. A patient has become disabled as a result of an automobile accident. The case manager has documented concerns about the patient's ability to perform instrumental activities of daily living. Based on your knowledge, what activities are included in this listing?

Exercise 2

Virtual Hospital Activity

45 minutes

- Sign in to work at Pacific View Regional Hospital on the Medical-Surgical Floor for Period of Care 1. (*Note:* If you are already in the virtual hospital from a previous exercise, click on **Leave the Floor** and then on **Restart the Program** to get to the sign-in window.)
- From the Patient List, select Patricia Newman (Room 406).
- Click on **Get Report**.
- Click on **Go to Nurses' Station**.
- Click on **Chart** and select the chart for Room **406**.
- Click on and then review the **Nursing Admission** and **History and Physical**.

1. What is Patricia Newman's chief complaint at the time of admission?

2. According to Patricia Newman's past medical history, she has a history of several medical disorders. Listed below are her primary medical diagnoses. Prioritize these disorders in order of importance for this hospital admission.

Medical Diagnosis	Priority
_____ Tobacco use	a. 1st
_____ Emphysema	b. 2nd
_____ Pneumonia	c. 3rd
_____ Osteoporosis	d. 4th
_____ Hypertension	e. 5th

3. During the nursing admission, Patricia Newman described her health as "not very good." This is an example of:
   a. objective data.
   b. back channeling.
   c. defining characteristics.
   d. subjective data.

 • Click on **Return to Nurses' Station**.
   • Click on **406** at the bottom of the screen.
   • Review the Initial Observations.

4. Based on your knowledge of Patricia Newman's condition and a review of the Initial Observations, which of the following tasks should the nurse perform first after entering the room?
   a. Assess patient's vital signs.
   b. Check patient's arm band for identification.
   c. Assess patient's neurologic status.
   d. Determine patient's chief concern at this time.

• Click on **Patient Care** and then on **Nurse-Client Interactions**.
   • Select and view the video titled **0730: Prioritizing Interventions**. (*Note:* Check the virtual clock to see whether enough time has elapsed. You can use the fast-forward feature to advance the time by 2-minute intervals if the video is not yet available. Then click again on **Patient Care** and on **Nurse-Client Interactions** to refresh the screen.)

5. Based on the video, what has been identified as the priority intervention by the nurse?

6. Based on the video, what concern does Patricia Newman have? Is this concern shared by the nurse?

7. Critique the nurse-patient interaction in the video. What strengths does the nurse display in her interaction with Patricia Newman?

8. What action should the nurse take after receiving report?
   a. Discuss the plan of care for the day with the patient.
   b. Validate patient's pulmonary status by conducting a physical examination.
   c. Begin instruction on breathing exercises.
   d. Call the physician to review data from the report.

9. During the physical assessment, you are able to review Patricia Newman's cardiovascular and respiratory status. What other sources of data might you use to support your findings?

10. After gathering data from the physical assessment to further define potential problem areas, the following issues are identified. Prioritize the potential problems in order of importance.

Potential Problems	Priority
_____ Nutritional intake	a. 1st
_____ Oxygenation	b. 2nd
_____ Health promotion habits	c. 3rd
_____ Reduced energy level	d. 4th

11. Data clusters are sets of signs or symptoms that are grouped together logically. Match each sign or symptom with its appropriate data cluster category.

Sign or Symptom	**Category of Data Cluster**
_____ PaO$_2$ below normal	a. Respiratory/oxygenation
_____ Dyspnea on exertion	b. Reduced energy level
_____ Productive cough	
_____ Oxygen saturation 92%	
_____ Feels "too tired to do much"	
_____ Requires frequent rest periods	
_____ Respirations labored	

12. As you identify clusters of data, you begin to recognize patterns or trends. Data often contain defining characteristics, or criteria, for nursing diagnoses. Listed below are three nursing diagnoses with defining characteristics. Which of the diagnoses would likely apply to Patricia Newman? Select all that apply.

    _____ Ineffective Airway Clearance: Diminished breath sounds, dyspnea, adventitious breath sounds, ineffective cough, sputum production, changes in respiratory rate

    _____ Impaired Gas Exchange: Tachycardia, hypoxia, abnormal arterial blood gases, abnormal rate and depth of breathing, hypoxemia

    _____ Ineffective Breathing Pattern: Pursed-lip breathing, dyspnea, use of accessory muscles to breathe, respiratory rate higher than 24 per minute, altered chest excursion

➤ • Select and view the videos titled **0740: Evaluation: Response to Care** and **0750: Evaluation: Patient Teaching**. (*Note:* Check the virtual clock to see whether enough time has elapsed. You can use the fast-forward feature to advance the time by 2-minute intervals if the video is not yet available. Then click again on **Patient Care** and on **Nurse-Client Interactions** to refresh the screen.)

13. Consultation is based on the _____ approach.

14. Consultation increases the nurse's _____ about a problem.

15. The plan of care often requires input from a variety of disciplines. Consider Patricia Newman's needs. Which members of the health care team could provide useful input into the plan of care?

• Click on **Chart** and then on **406**.

  • Click on and then review the **Physician's Orders**, **Physician's Notes**, and **Consultations**.

16. A series of interventions are indicated to assist Patricia Newman in managing her impaired gas exchange problems. Match each intervention with its correct type. (*Hint:* Refer to your textbook if you need help identifying types of interventions.)

Interventions	Type
_____ Administer oxygen at 2 L per nasal cannula.	a. Nurse-initiated
_____ Instruct patient on how to perform pursed-lip breathing.	b. Physician-initiated
_____ Position patient with head of bed elevated to 45 degrees.	c. Collaborative
_____ Administer bronchodilator by a metered-dose inhaler (MDI).	
_____ Have the patient perform cascade coughing every 1 hour.	
_____ Encourage oral fluids of 3 L daily.	

17. A nurse caring for Patricia Newman performs the following activities. Which of these activities are examples of indirect care measures? Select all that apply.

  _____ Adjusts the oxygen flow meter to ensure that it runs correctly and checks condition of the tubing

  _____ Coaches Patricia Newman on the technique for performing a cascade cough

  _____ Documents the character of Patricia Newman's cough and ability to expectorate mucus

  _____ Consults with the respiratory therapist about Patricia Newman's use of an MDI

  _____ Administers intravenous (IV) fluid infusion

18. For each of the expected outcomes listed below and on the next page, write an evaluation measure.

  a. Patient's lungs will clear without crackles within 48 hours:

b. Patient's fluid intake will be 3 L every 24 hours:

c. Patient will perform pursed-lip breathing correctly within 24 hours:

d. Patient will experience less dyspnea while ambulating within 2 days:

LESSON 4 —————————————————

Communication with the Patient and Health Care Team

 Reading Assignment: Communication (Chapter 24)

Patients: Dorothy Grant, Obstetrics Floor, Room 201
Kathryn Doyle, Skilled Nursing Floor, Room 503

Objectives:

1. Describe the levels and corresponding uses of communication in nursing.
2. Describe the elements of the communication process.
3. Discuss behaviors and communication techniques that affect professional communication.
4. Identify factors that create barriers to communication.

Exercise 1

 Writing Activity

20 minutes

1. Identify the five levels of communication.

2. _____ are means of conveying and receiving messages through visual, auditory, and tactile senses.

3. When a nurse is discussing discharge instructions with a patient, the recommended amount of space between the nurse and patient is:
   a. 12 to 18 inches.
   b. 18 inches to 4 feet.
   c. 5 to 6 feet.
   d. at least 8 feet.

4. A therapeutic nurse-patient interaction is necessary to promote quality care. Which of the following elements foster a therapeutic nurse-patient relationship? Select all that apply.

   _____ Hugging

   _____ Sincerity

   _____ Empathy

   _____ Trustworthiness

   _____ Sympathy

   _____ False reassurance

   _____ Caring attitude

5. Discuss the importance of the use of silence when interacting with a patient.

6. When providing written communication to a visually impaired patient, it is necessary to use

   a font (typeface) that is at least _____ points or greater.

7. _____ conveys a sense of self-assurance and respect for the other person in the communication exchange.

8. _____ Offering false reassurance can be therapeutic if the patient has only a narrow margin of hope. (True/False)

9. _____ When considering gender differences related to communication patterns, a nurse knows that men are more likely to address issues more directly than women. (True/False)

10. Which of the following statements best represents a defensive response?
    a. "I know that pain medication was effective."
    b. "You seem different today."
    c. "You have really had such a hard time getting by lately."
    d. "The care you are getting is the best anywhere."

Exercise 2

 Virtual Hospital Activity

 30 minutes

- Sign in to work at Pacific View Regional Hospital on the Obstetrics Floor for Period of Care 2. (*Note:* If you are already in the virtual hospital from a previous exercise, click on **Leave the Floor** and then on **Restart the Program** to get to the sign-in window.)
- From the Patient List, select Dorothy Grant (Room 201).
- Click on **Get Report**.
- Click on **Go to Nurses' Station**.
- Click on **Chart** and then on **201**.
- Click on and then review the **Nursing Admission** and **History and Physical**.

1. Why has Dorothy Grant been admitted to the hospital?

2. The change-of-shift report indicates Dorothy Grant has been anxious and crying. As you prepare to go to her room, what might you consider in your initial communication approach?

3. During the working phase of the relationship between the nurse and Dorothy Grant, what activities should take place? Select all that apply.

    _____ Encourage her to engage in self-exploration.

    _____ Identify a location and setting for interacting with her.

    _____ Evaluate goal achievement.

    _____ Provide information needed to understand and change potential problematic behaviors.

    _____ Encourage the patient to seek help.

    _____ Clarify the role of the nurse.

4. Active listening will be an important communication technique as you talk with Dorothy Grant. There are several nonverbal skills that facilitate attentive listening. Below, identify these techniques by using the SOLER mnemonic device.

S:

O:

L:

E:

R:

➤ • Click on **Return to Nurses' Station**.
   • Click on **201** at the bottom of the screen.
   • Review the Initial Observations.
   • Click on **Patient Care** and then on **Nurse-Client Interactions**.
   • Select and view the video titled **1115: Nurse-Patient Communication**. (*Note:* Check the virtual clock to see whether enough time has elapsed. You can use the fast-forward feature to advance the time by 2-minute intervals if the video is not yet available. Then click again on **Patient Care** and on **Nurse-Client Interactions** to refresh the screen.)

5. The first question presented to Dorothy Grant by the nurse was a(n)

   _____ question.

6. As you observe the nurse-patient interaction, select the listening techniques the nurse used from the list below. Select all that apply.

   _____   Sit facing the patient.

   _____   Use an open posture.

   _____   Lean toward the patient.

   _____   Establish/maintain eye contact.

   _____   Relax.

7. The nurse tells Dorothy Grant, "Right now, your first priority is your well-being and the well-being of your baby." This is an example of what therapeutic technique?
   a. Empathy
   b. Sharing hope
   c. Providing information
   d. Paraphrasing

8. When talking with Dorothy Grant, which of the following questions/statements would be most therapeutic?
   a. "Tell me about your relationship with your husband."
   b. "Can you tell me why you have stayed in such an abusive relationship?"
   c. "Let's get some rest now and later we can talk about your relationship."
   d. "I imagine your pregnancy has caused stress to your relationship."

9. During the interaction, Dorothy Grant reports that although her sister is supportive, her parents "act as if nothing is going on." The nurse responds by stating, "That must be so frustrating." What type of communication technique is being used in this incidence?
   a. Sympathy
   b. Empathy
   c. Channeling
   d. Restatement

10. During the video interaction between Dorothy Grant and the nurse, which of the following zones of personal space is being used?
    a. Public zone
    b. Personal zone
    c. Intimate zone
    d. Social zone

Exercise 3

 Virtual Hospital Activity

 30 minutes

- Sign in to work at Pacific View Regional Hospital on the Skilled Nursing Floor for Period of Care 1. (*Note:* If you are already in the virtual hospital from a previous exercise, click on **Leave the Floor** and then on **Restart the Program** to get to the sign-in window.)
- From the Patient List, select Kathryn Doyle (Room 503).
- Click on **Get Report**.
- Click on **Go to Nurses' Station**.
- Click on **Chart** and then on **503**.
- Click on **Nursing Admission** and **History and Physical**; review the records.

1. Why has Kathryn Doyle been admitted to the hospital?

2. What are Kathryn Doyle's primary concerns and needs?

→ • Click on **Return to Nurses' Station**.
   • Click on **503** at the bottom of your screen.
   • Review the Initial Observations.
   • Click on **Patient Care** and then on **Nurse-Client Interactions**.
   • Select and view the video titled **0730: Assessment—Biopsychosocial**. (*Note:* Check the virtual clock to see whether enough time has elapsed. You can use the fast-forward feature to advance the time by 2-minute intervals if the video is not yet available. Then click again on **Patient Care** and on **Nurse-Client Interactions** to refresh the screen.)

3. During the interaction, the nurse asks Kathryn Doyle how she is feeling. The manner in

   which the question is phrased is a(n) _____
   question.

4. In response to Kathryn Doyle's complaints about how she is feeling, the nurse's verbal behaviors demonstrate which of the following communication techniques?
   a. Sympathy
   b. Approval
   c. Defensiveness
   d. Passiveness
   e. Aggressiveness

5. Review the behaviors exhibited by Kathryn Doyle. Comment on her voice, tone, and gestures.

6. In the absence of active nonverbal behaviors, eye contact can provide a great deal of information about the patient. What information can be gleaned from eye contact?

• Review the same video interaction again (0730: Assessment—Biopsychosocial).

7. The nurse asks Kathryn Doyle, "Do you have any concerns you would like to talk about?" What are the limitations of this particular question posed by the nurse?

8. During this interaction, Kathryn Doyle refers to her concerns about being discharged. She states, "Well, I've been thinking of going home and wondering just what it's going to be like." Below, write an appropriate response to the patient's concern for each of the therapeutic communication techniques listed.

Paraphrasing

Sharing observation

Clarifying

• Select and view the video titled **0733: Planning—Fact Finding**. (*Note:* Check the virtual clock to see whether enough time has elapsed. You can use the fast-forward feature to advance the time by 2-minute intervals if the video is not yet available. Then click again on **Patient Care** and on **Nurse-Client Interactions** to refresh the screen.)

9. When discussing Kathryn Doyle's weight loss, the nurse responds by saying, "Oh, why do you think that is?" What type of response is this?
   a. Asking for an explanation
   b. Clarifying
   c. Focusing
   d. Automatic response

10. Was the nursing response in the above question the best option? Why or why not?

• Select and view the video titled **0740: Planning for Care**. (*Note:* Check the virtual clock to see whether enough time has elapsed. You can use the fast-forward feature to advance the time by 2-minute intervals if the video is not yet available. Then click again on **Patient Care** and on **Nurse-Client Interactions** to refresh the screen.)

11. During the interaction, the nurse uses touch. What is being conveyed by the nurse's touch?

Patient Teaching in Practice

 Reading Assignment: Patient Education (Chapter 25)

Patient: Patricia Newman, Medical-Surgical Floor, Room 406

Objectives:

1. Identify the role of the nurse in patient education.
2. Identify the purposes of patient education.
3. Review communication principles when providing patient education.
4. Identify learning principles.

Exercise 1

 Writing Activity

🕐 20 minutes

1. Which of the following statements concerning patient education is correct? Select all that apply.

   _____ Patient teaching can reduce the reoccurrences of illness.

   _____ Patient teaching increases the overall costs associated with hospitalization.

   _____ Patient teaching promotes the patient's ability to exert control over his or her own care.

   _____ Patient teaching can reduce the need for costly medical procedures.

2. _____ can best be defined as an interactive process that promotes learning.

3. The purposeful acquisition of new knowledge, attitudes, behaviors, and skills is referred to

   as _____.

4. An individual's perceived ability to successfully complete a task refers to the concept of

   _____.

5. List the three domains of learning.

6. A nurse is planning to allow a patient the opportunity to select her own diet and monitor glucose levels for a 12-hour period. Which of the following approaches to learning is being demonstrated by this nurse?
   a. Participating
   b. Entrusting
   c. Reinforcing
   d. Role modeling

7. A nurse is planning to use an analogy to teach a patient about the manifestations associated with premenstrual syndrome. Which of the following concepts must be incorporated into this method of instruction? Select all that apply.

   _____ Familiarity with the material being presented

   _____ Pamphlets and diagrams regarding the disorder

   _____ Knowledge of the patient's background

   _____ Use of a simple and clear analogy

8. You are preparing to provide education to an adolescent concerning newly prescribed medications. Which of the following methods will be most effective?
   a. Using photo books to relay the information
   b. Focusing on how the medication will promote the adolescent's strength
   c. Providing the education in a short session
   d. Viewing the education session as a collaborative activity

9. What factors make for the "ideal setting" when teaching a patient? Consider additional factors that should be taken into consideration when teaching a group of patients.

10. _____ is a force that acts on or within a person to cause a person to behave in a particular way.

Exercise 2

Virtual Hospital Activity

30 minutes

- Sign in to work at Pacific View Regional Hospital on the Medical-Surgical Floor for Period of Care 1. (*Note:* If you are already in the virtual hospital from a previous exercise, click on **Leave the Floor** and then on **Restart the Program** to get to the sign-in window.)
- From the Patient List, select Patricia Newman (Room 406).
- Click on **Get Report**.
- Click on **Go to Nurses' Station**.
- Click on **Chart** and then on **406**.
- Click on **Nursing Admission**; review the record.

1. Why has Patricia Newman been admitted to the hospital?

2. Based on the information you have read in the chart, list four of Patricia Newman's learning needs.

3. Identify family members and health care providers who should be included in the teaching being provided to Patricia Newman.

4. Consider Patricia Newman's learning needs. Below, match the learning domains with her specific learning needs.

Learning Need	**Learning Domain**
_____ Adoption of health promotion behaviors	a. Cognitive
_____ Understanding the benefits of not smoking	b. Affective
_____ Proper use of a metered-dose inhaler (MDI)	c. Psychomotor
_____ Being able to count caloric intake each day	

- Click on **Return to Nurses' Station**.
- Click on **406** at the bottom of your screen.
- Review the Initial Observations.
- Click on **Patient Care** and then on **Nurse-Client Interactions**.
- Select and view the videos titled **0730: Prioritizing Interventions** and **0740: Evaluation— Response to Care**. (*Note:* Check the virtual clock to see whether enough time has elapsed. You can use the fast-forward feature to advance the time by 2-minute intervals if the video is not yet available. Then click again on **Patient Care** and on **Nurse-Client Interactions** to refresh the screen.)

5. Nurses often combine teaching with daily patient care activities. During the videos, what teaching is being done by the nurse?

6. Discuss the advantages of providing education to patients while performing routine nursing care.

7. During the video interaction, Patricia Newman displays acceptance of her condition and related limitations. What are the implications for the nurse when planning future education to her?
   a. Let the patient know you are available for discussion
   b. Teach only in the present tense
   c. Encourage expression of feelings
   d. Focus on teaching about future skills and knowledge needed

 8. The respiratory therapist will be working with Patricia Newman on the use of a peak flow meter as a means to detect changes in her airway resistance. (*Study Tip:* Review pulmonary diagnostic studies in your textbook.) Select the factors that should be assessed in regard to Patricia Newman's ability to learn. Select all that apply.

_____ Distracters in the room during demonstration of the meter

_____ Coordination and endurance to hold meter and perform breathing maneuver

_____ Patient's belief in the need to improve lung function

_____ Patient's learning style preference

9. When developing the plan of care, a nurse knows that which of the following learning objectives regarding teaching Patricia Newman on the use of a peak flow meter is most appropriate?
   a. The patient will be able to demonstrate the correct use of the peak flow meter in 2 days.
   b. The nurse will provide education to the patient concerning the use of the peak flow meter before discharge.
   c. The peak flow meter will be used by the patient at the next period of administration.
   d. The patient will understand the use of the peak flow meter.

 • Click on **Chart** and then on **406**.
   • Click on **Patient Education** and review.

10. For each of the learning goals listed on Patricia Newman's teaching plan, critique and explain below how the goal or objective could be written more clearly.

Patient will comply with dietary recommendations.

Patient will understand rationale and perform pursed-lip breathing.

Patient will demonstrate correct use of MDI.

11. When planning to teach Patricia Newman on the use of the peak flow meter, the nurse should include which of the following in the discussion? Select all that apply.

_____ Classification of the medication

_____ Rationale for use of the medication

_____ Steps needed to use the meter

_____ Prognosis for the patient with emphysema

_____ Timing of the use of the meter

→ • Click on **Return to Room 406**.
  • Click on **Patient Care** and then on **Nurse-Client Interactions**.
  • Select and view the video titled **0750: Evaluation—Patient Teaching**. (*Note:* Check the virtual clock to see whether enough time has elapsed. You can use the fast-forward feature to advance the time by 2-minute intervals if the video is not yet available. Then click again on **Patient Care** and on **Nurse-Client Interactions** to refresh the screen.)

12. During the video interaction, the nurse missed an opportunity to evaluate Patricia Newman's learning. What should the nurse have done?

13. _____ Mastery of a task, such as self-administration of an inhaler, is often based on the need for achievement. (True/False)

14. There are three primary purposes of patient education. Match each of the following education topics with its correct purpose.

Education Topic	**Purpose**
_____ Walking more frequently at longer intervals	a. Health promotion
_____ Quitting smoking	b. Health restoration
_____ Rationale for use and correct schedule of inhaler	c. Coping with impaired function
_____ Benefit of a flu shot	
_____ Administration of home oxygen	

15. Patricia Newman will be receiving instruction on a number of topics. Match each of the following teaching topics with the appropriate instructional method.

Instructional Method	**Teaching Topic**
_____ Simulation	a. Pursed-lip breathing
_____ Demonstration	b. Side effects of medication
_____ Role playing	c. Planning a dinner high in protein
_____ One-to-one discussion	d. Learning to say no when a friend offers a cigarette
_____ Use of analogies	e. Explaining how high blood pressure creates an effect similar to forcing water through a constricted hose

16. Listed below are instructional topics relating to Patricia Newman's needs. For each topic, identify the best evaluation method.

Self-administration of an MDI

Patient's ability to increase her walking distance

Patient's compliance with a high-calorie diet

Documentation Principles

 Reading Assignment: Documentation and Informatics (Chapter 26)

Patients: Pablo Rodriguez, Medical-Surgical Floor, Room 405
Kathryn Doyle, Skilled Nursing Floor, Room 503

Objectives:

1. Identify the purpose of medical records.
2. Describe the documentation responsibilities of nurses.
3. Recognize the different types of documentation used by nurses.
4. Critique the quality of a change-of-shift report.

Exercise 1

 Writing Activity

30 minutes

1. It is vital that every member of the health care team follow the rules and regulations imposed by HIPAA. What do the initials HIPAA stand for?

   H:

   I:

   P:

   A:

   A:

2. What are the purposes of documentation?

3. A newly hired graduate nurse is advised that the facility uses PIE charting. Which of the following statements by the graduate nurse indicates the need for further clarification?
   a. "PIE charting is focused charting."
   b. "PIE charting is problem-oriented."
   c. "PIE charting is nursing-focused."
   d. "PIE charting does not provide an assessment in the narrative data recorded."

4. A nurse who has already gone home calls back to the nursing unit and reports that she has forgotten to note the patient's activity during her shift. Which of the following is the appropriate action by the nurse who is currently on the unit?
   a. Agree to note the patient's activities and sign the other nurse's signature.
   b. Contact the nursing supervisor.
   c. Advise the nurse that his or her concerns will be passed along but that the information will not be documented in his or her absence.
   d. Refuse to become involved.

5. When documenting a patient treatment, a nurse realizes he made an error when recording information. Which of the following actions by the nurse is most appropriate?
   a. Erase the information that was recorded in error.
   b. Obtain a new flow sheet and start the page over.
   c. Use a permanent marker and completely cover the information recorded in error.
   d. Call the nursing supervisor.
   e. Neatly draw a single line through the error and then add the correct information.

6. Identify the elements of SOAP charting.

S:

O:

A:

P:

7. A patient's chart has a separate section for each discipline when _____ records are used.

8. A facility uses DAR charting. The nurse correctly recognizes that "A" represents which of the following?
   a. Assessment
   b. Activity
   c. Action
   d. Adaptation

9. _____ When giving a transfer report, the nurse should include a discussion of any assessment that should be completed shortly after the transfer. (True/False)

10. _____ It is appropriate for the unit secretary to take report from another care unit when the nurse is occupied with other patients. (True/False)

11. What information can the nurse expect to find in the Kardex? Select all that apply.

_____   Primary medical diagnosis

_____   Scheduled medications

_____   Nursing care plan

_____   Family medical history

_____   Emergency contact information

12. What is the purpose of nursing informatics?

Exercise 2

 Virtual Hospital Activity

30 minutes

- Sign in to work at Pacific View Regional Hospital on the Skilled Nursing Floor for Period of Care 1. (*Note:* If you are already in the virtual hospital from a previous exercise, click on **Leave the Floor** and then on **Restart the Program** to get to the sign-in window.)
- From the Patient List, select Kathryn Doyle (Room 503).
- Click on **Get Report**.
- Click on **Go to Nurses' Station**.
- Click on **503** at the bottom of the screen.
- Review the Initial Observations.
- Click on **Take Vital Signs**.

1. Based on the report received, what are the greatest priorities to address during the initial interaction with Kathryn Doyle?

2. Based on the Initial Observations and assessment of vital signs, was the report accurate? Explain.

3. The report summary indicates that Kathryn Doyle received oxycodone and acetaminophen for pain in the left hip. Place an X next to each of the following criteria that should have been included in the description of pain. Select all that apply.

_____ Condition of the right hip

_____ Onset of pain

_____ Severity of pain

_____ Effectiveness of pain medication

_____ Factors that worsen pain

_____ Duration of pain

→ • Click on **Chart** and then on **503**.
  • Click on **Nurse's Notes** and review the entries for Tuesday and Wednesday.

4. The type of charting being used by Pacific View Regional Hospital, as demonstrated in the

   Nurse's Notes, is _____.

5. _____ Kathryn Doyle's chart is an example of a problem-oriented medical record (POMR). (True/False)

6. Review the Nurse's Notes entered for Wednesday at 0715. Are there any elements of the entry that you feel could be better stated? Which? Why?

→ • Now, click on **Return to Room 503**.
  • Click on **EPR** and **Login**.
  • Select **503** from the Patient drop-down menu and **Vital Signs** from the Category drop-down menu.

7. Which of the following terms can best be used to describe the type of documentation represented by the EPR?
   a. Flow sheet
   b. Database
   c. Focus charting
   d. SOAP charting

8. What are the advantages of the type of charting represented by the EPR?

 • Click on **Exit EPR**.
   • Click on **Chart** and then on **503**.
   • Click on **History and Physical**, **Nursing Admission**, and **Nurse's Notes** and review the records. Specifically review the Nurse's Notes for Wed 0555.

9. If Kathryn Doyle's health care team were using a critical pathway, her wound infection, anemia, and uncontrolled pain would be considered unexpected outcomes and would be

   called _____.

10. The entry of 0555 represents what time in standard notation?
    a. 5:55 p.m.
    b. 12:05 a.m.
    c. 5:55 a.m.
    d. 12:55 p.m.

11. Rewrite the narrative note for 0555 in a PIE format.

12. What information could have been provided by the nurse to make the 0555 narrative note more complete in regard to Kathryn Doyle's problems with pain management?

→ • Click on **Physician's Orders**.
  • Review the orders received on Tuesday at 1530.

13. The order for an evaluation by a psychiatric nurse was received via

   _____.

14. Discuss the steps needed when encountering the type of order identified in the preceding question.

15. Has the nursing staff correctly handled the telephone order noted at 0555 on Tuesday?

→ • Click on **Nursing Admission** and review the record.

16. Medical records serve several purposes. Match each application of information from Kathryn Doyle's record with its correct purpose.

Application

_____ Data show that Kathryn Doyle's allergy history was entered.

_____ A review of Kathryn Doyle's self-perception helps demonstrate factors that influence a person's body image.

_____ Kathryn Doyle's assessment shows she is sleeping poorly, tires easily, and receives no regular exercise.

_____ Kathryn Doyle is age 79. She has a history of osteoporosis, she fell at home, and she takes calcium daily.

Purpose

a. Communication of patient problem

b. Use of records to research character-istics of patients who have had hip surgery

c. Auditing of chart for regulatory requirements

d. Education for understanding the nature of nursing concepts

17. When Kathryn Doyle is ready for discharge, which of the following will be included in the discharge summary? Select all that apply.

_____ Patient's prognosis

_____ Listing of medications taken during the hospitalization

_____ Narrative of diagnostic test results performed during the hospitalization

_____ Teaching needs

_____ Plans for rehabilitation

18. A(n) _____ is a tool that can be used to allow for the various disciplines to participate in Kathryn Doyle's plan of care.

Exercise 3

Virtual Hospital Activity

30 minutes

- Sign in to work at Pacific View Regional Hospital on the Medical-Surgical Floor for Period of Care 1. (*Note:* If you are already in the virtual hospital from a previous exercise, click on **Leave the Floor** and then on **Restart the Program** to get to the sign-in window.)
- From the Patient List, select Pablo Rodriguez (Room 405).
- Click on **Get Report**.

1. Why has Pablo Rodriguez been admitted to the hospital?

2. Based on the clinical report, what concerns are currently of the highest priority for Pablo Rodriguez?

3. The clinical report is a reflection of the information typically shared between nurses during the change-of-shift report. One of the advantages of oral reports is the ability to ask questions. After reviewing the report for Pablo Rodriguez, list three questions you might ask the night nurse.

4. Which of the following would be appropriate for the nurse to do during the change-of-shift report? Select all that apply.

_____ Describe the basic steps of how the patient uses a PCA.

_____ Describe objective measures such as "oxygen at 3 liters."

_____ Evaluate the result of morphine when given for pain in nodules.

_____ Preview the patient's age, occupation, and education.

_____ Identify and explain the patient's immediate priorities of care.

 • Click on **Go to Nurses' Station**.
 • Click on **405** at the bottom of the screen.
 • Click on **Patient Care** and then on **Nurse-Client Interactions**.
 • Select and view the video titled **0730: Symptom Management**. (*Note:* Check the virtual clock to see whether enough time has elapsed. You can use the fast-forward feature to advance the time by 2-minute intervals if the video is not yet available. Then click again on **Patient Care** and on **Nurse-Client Interactions** to refresh the screen.)

5. _____ Pablo Rodriguez voices considerable anxiety about telling his children about his feelings. In order to reduce his anxiety and improve his condition, the nurse may relay these concerns to the family. (True/False)

 • Click on **Initial Observations**; review the note.
 • Click on **Patient Care** and then on **Nurse-Client Interactions**.
 • Select and view the video titled **0735: Patient Perceptions**. (*Note:* Check the virtual clock to see whether enough time has elapsed. You can use the fast-forward feature to advance the time by 2-minute intervals if the video is not yet available. Then click again on **Patient Care** and on **Nurse-Client Interactions** to refresh the screen.)

6. Discuss differences between the clinical report and the Initial Observations at 0730.

7. Based on the video you just observed, write a DAR note describing the interaction with Pablo Rodriguez.

➡ • Click on **Patient Care** and then on **Physical Assessment**.
  • Complete a systems assessment by clicking on the body system categories (yellow buttons) and body system subcategories (green buttons).

8. If a charting-by-exception approach were to be employed, which of the following body systems would be discussed in the progress notes? Select all that apply.

_____   Neurologic

_____   Cardiovascular

_____   Pulmonary

_____   Integumentary

_____   Gastrointestinal

_____   Urologic

_____   Reproductive

9. Pablo Rodriguez has an IV. What information should be included in the documentation regarding the IV?

10. Pablo Rodriguez has vomited his medications. Which of the following statements should the nurse document about the incident?
   a. The patient vomited this morning.
   b. The patient vomited 100 mL of green emesis.
   c. The patient reports vomiting this morning.
   d. Continued vomiting by patient noted.

11. The nurse is preparing to administer medications prescribed for Pablo Rodriguez's nausea. Which of the following will be documented on the patient's MAR? Select all that apply.

   _____ Time of administration

   _____ Route of administration

   _____ Site of administration

   _____ Therapeutic effect of medication

   _____ Patient's last episode of emesis

   _____ Initials of nurse administering the medication

LESSON **7**

Self-Concept

 Reading Assignment: Self-Concept (Chapter 33)

Patients: Dorothy Grant, Obstetrics Floor, Room 201
Harry George, Medical-Surgical Floor, Room 401

Objectives:

1. Identify the components of self-concept.
2. Describe stressors that affect the self-concept of two patients.
3. Discuss the influence of a nurse's behavior on a patients' self-concept.
4. Apply the critical thinking model to the assessment of a patient's self-concept.
5. Develop a concept map for a case study patient with self-concept alterations.
6. Describe the nursing diagnostic process for a patient with alterations in self-concept.
7. Identify interventions useful in the promotion of self-concept.

Exercise 1

 Writing Activity

15 minutes

1. Identify three self-concept issues that a nurse should clarify about himself or herself when caring for patients.

2. A nurse is interacting with a hospitalized patient. Which of the following behaviors signals a potentially negative alteration in self-concept? Select all that apply.

   _____ The patient is aggressively seeking information about treatment options.

   _____ The patient passively listens to information about planned diagnostic testing.

   _____ The patient is critical about the care being received thus far.

   _____ The patient repeatedly apologizes for asking questions of the health care team.

   _____ The patient takes notes about the information being provided by the nurse.

3. Key indicators of a patient's self-concept can be _____ behaviors.

4. A nurse is caring for an 8-year-old child. When evaluating the child, the nurse knows that which of the following behaviors by the child indicates positive progression through the age-appropriate developmental stage?
   a. Accepts body changes
   b. Attempts to put information obtained from parents and teachers to use
   c. Begins to communicate likes and dislikes
   d. Has positive feelings about self

5. Which of the following developmental tasks must be accomplished by a 75-year-old patient?
   a. Ego integrity versus despair
   b. Intimacy versus isolation
   c. Industry versus inferiority
   d. Initiative versus guilt

6. _____ Self-esteem is highest in childhood. (True/False)

7. _____ Concerns with body image tend not to plague men. (True/False)

Exercise 2

 Virtual Hospital Activity

 30 minutes

- Sign in to work at Pacific View Regional Hospital on the Medical-Surgical Floor for Period of Care 3. (*Note:* If you are already in the virtual hospital from a previous exercise, click on **Leave the Floor** and then on **Restart the Program** to get to the sign-in window.)
- From the Patient List, select Harry George (Room 401).
- Click on **Get Report**.
- Click on **Go to Nurses' Station**.
- Click on **Chart** and then on **401**.
- Click on **Nursing Admission** and **History and Physical**; review the records.

1. Self-concept is always changing and developing. Which of the following factors have affected Harry George's self-concept since his motorcycle accident 4 years ago? Select all that apply.

   _____ Sense of competency

   _____ Perceived reaction of others to his body

   _____ Employment-related identity

   _____ Perceptions of events that have affected self

   _____ Racial identity

   _____ Self-expectations

2. Explain how the loss of employment has likely affected Harry George's self-concept.

3. Of the following developmental stages of life described by Erik Erikson, which is most likely disrupted in the case of Harry George?
   a. Integrity versus despair
   b. Industry versus inferiority
   c. Initiative versus guilt
   d. Generativity versus self-absorption

➔ • Now click on **Consultations** and **Mental Health**; review the Psychiatric Consult and Mental Health record.

4. A self-concept stressor threatens a person's identity, body image, and role performance. Match the stressors experienced by Harry George with the appropriate self-concept category.

Harry George's Stressors	Self-Concept Categories
_____ Impotence	a. Body image
_____ Loss of role as husband	b. Identity
_____ Emotional depression	c. Role performance
_____ Failure to maintain personal grooming	
_____ Job loss	
_____ Chronic wound	
_____ Seen as a public nuisance	

5. The expectations of family and friends on how Harry George should have behaved immediately following his injury would be described as a(n) _____ role.

6. Harry George's _____ image involves attitudes he has about his appearance, impotence, and the effects of his diabetes.

7. Harry George's emotional appraisal of himself as a "loser" is a form of self-evaluation described as _____-esteem.

8. Harry George's _____ performance is the way in which he perceives his ability to be competent as a parent.

9. Harry George is a complex case. Given the nursing diagnoses of Chronic Low Self-Esteem, Social Isolation, and Ineffective Coping, which would likely be your priority? Explain.

Exercise 3

Virtual Hospital Activity

30 minutes

- Sign in to work at Pacific View Regional Hospital on the Obstetrics Floor for Period of Care 1. (*Note:* If you are already in the virtual hospital from a previous exercise, click on **Leave the Floor** and then on **Restart the Program** to get to the sign-in window.)
- From the Patient List, select Dorothy Grant (Room 201).
- Click on **Get Report**.
- Click on **Go to Nurses' Station**.
- Click on **Chart** and then on **201**.
- Click on **History and Physical** and **Nursing Admission**; review the records.

1. Provide a brief overview of Dorothy Grant and the reason for her hospital admission.

2. As a victim of abuse, Dorothy Grant faces many factors that threaten her self-concept. Her concern for her unborn baby and her other children creates stress on her ability to function as a wife and mother. Application of critical thinking will ensure a more comprehensive assessment of this patient's situation. Listed below are specific critical thinking factors that apply to Dorothy Grant's situation. Use these letters to complete the critical thinking assessment diagram (write each letter on a line under its proper category.

Knowledge

1. _____

2. _____

3. _____

Experience

Assessment of Self-Concept

Standards

4. _____

5. _____

6. _____

7. _____

Attitudes

8. _____

9. _____

Critical Thinking Factors

a. If, as a parent, you have ever believed your children were at risk, consider your own feelings in that regard.

b. Say to Dorothy Grant, "You said you want to be a good mother. Tell me what you mean by that."

c. Review concepts on domestic violence.

d. While caring for Dorothy Grant, apply what you have learned in caring for other victims of abuse.

e. While assessing Dorothy Grant, reinforce that any decisions about getting help to leave her husband will be her decisions only.

f. Consider concepts about self-esteem as you assess Dorothy Grant's needs.

g. Ask Dorothy Grant to tell her story by saying, "Tell me how your relationship with your husband has changed since you first married."

h. Ask the patient if you can talk with her sister about her relationship with her children.

i. Apply principles of communication and caring while establishing a therapeutic relationship with Dorothy Grant.

 • Click on **Return to Nurses' Station**.

• Click on **Leave the Floor**; then click on **Restart the Program**.

• Sign in to work at Pacific View Regional Hospital on the Obstetrics Floor for Period of Care 3.

• From the Patient List, select Dorothy Grant (Room 201).

• Click on **Get Report**.

• Click on **Go to Nurses' Station**.

- Click on **201** at the bottom of screen.
- Click on **Patient Care** and then on **Nurse-Client Interactions**.
- Select and view the video titled **1500: Managing Preterm Labor**. (*Note:* Check the virtual clock to see whether enough time has elapsed. You can use the fast-forward feature to advance the time by 2-minute intervals if the video is not yet available Then click again on **Patient Care** and on **Nurse-Client Interactions** to refresh the screen.)

3. List three nursing behaviors observed during the video interaction that reflect the nurse's acceptance of Dorothy Grant.

- Click on **Chart**; then click on **201**.
- Select **Consultations**. Review the Psychiatric Consult and Social Work Consult.

4. The information from Dorothy Grant's medical record provides considerable information about her health problems. Fill in the missing pieces of the diagnostic process chart below. (*Hint:* Locations of missing pieces are numbered 1 through 4 in the chart.)

Assessment Activities	Defining Characteristics	Nursing Diagnosis
Observe patient's nonverbal behaviors.	During admission patient is seen crying and wringing her hands.	4.
Observe patient's self-report of situation.	Patient reports being scared.	
Ask patient about decisions made or test her ability to problem-solve.	Patient reports that decisions are deferred to her husband.	
1.	Patient states she is unable to please husband.	Situational low self-esteem
2.	"I'm scared—what am I going to do?"	
Ask patient to describe how she feels about situation.	3.	

5. For the diagnosis of Situational Low Self-Esteem, list three interventions you would plan for Dorothy Grant and give a rationale for each.

The Experience of Loss, Death, and Grief: Nursing Interventions to Support Coping

Reading Assignment: Planning Nursing Care (Chapter 18, pages 248-249)
The Experience of Loss, Death, and Grief (Chapter 36)
Stress and Coping (Chapter 37)

Patients: Harry George, Medical-Surgical Floor, Room 401
Goro Oishi, Skilled Nursing Floor, Room 505

Objectives:

1. Describe types of loss.
2. Identify characteristics of a person experiencing grief.
3. Explain the relationship between loss and stress.
4. Describe the coping mechanisms used by two patients.
5. Describe the role of hope when providing support for a patient experiencing grief.
6. Describe principles of palliative care.
7. Identify applicable nursing diagnoses to a patient requiring palliative care.

Exercise 1

 Writing Activity

 10 minutes

1. A nurse is caring for a patient who embraces the traditional Chinese beliefs about death and dying. The nurse should recognize which of the following?
   a. Burial should occur within 24 hours after the death.
   b. Organ donation is viewed as a desirable service to perform for others.
   c. Religious rituals are important at the time of death.
   d. Death is viewed as a negative event.

2. Self-destructive or maladaptive behavior, obsessions, or psychiatric disorders are

   characteristic of a(n) _____ grief response.

3. According to Bowlby's phases of mourning, the phase of

   _____ arouses emotional outbursts and acute distress.

4. _____ helps patients to maintain anticipation of a continued good.

Exercise 2

Virtual Hospital Activity

30 minutes

- Sign in to work at Pacific View Regional Hospital on the Skilled Nursing Floor for Period of Care 1. (*Note:* If you are already in the virtual hospital from a previous exercise, click on **Leave the Floor** and then on **Restart the Program** to get to the sign-in window.)
- From the Patient List, select Goro Oishi (Room 505).
- Click on **Get Report**; review the report and then click on **Go to Nurses' Station**.
- Click on **Chart** and then on **505**.
- Click on **History and Physical** and on the **Nursing Admission**. Review the records.

1. Goro Oishi has been admitted for hospice care. Which of the following describe the components or features of a hospice care program? Select all that apply.

   _____ Provides treatment of terminal illnesses

   _____ Focuses on symptom control

   _____ Utilizes interdisciplinary care team approach

   _____ Sets goals to exclusively meet the patient's family's desires

   _____ Coordinates home care services

2. What factors in the History and Physical indicate that Goro Oishi might have experienced a perceived loss in the months before his stroke?

3. What is the significance of this type of loss? (*Hint:* See page 709 in your textbook.)

4. How did Goro Oishi choose to cope with his loss?

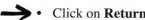 • Click on the **Physician's Notes** and on the **Nurse's Notes**. Review the records.

5. The notes state that Goro Oishi's family feels conflicted about whether or not to initiate enteral feeding. Which stages of grief might the family be experiencing at this time? Select all that apply.

_____ Adjusting to the environment without the deceased

_____ Reorganization

_____ Denial

_____ Bargaining

_____ Emotionally relocating the deceased

• Click on **Return to Nurses' Station**.
• Click on **505** at the bottom of the screen.
• Read the Initial Observations.
• Click on **Patient Care** and then on **Nurse-Client Interactions**.
• One at a time, select and view the following three videos: **0735: Assessment—Family**; **0750: Family Conflict—Plan of Care**; and **0755: Death—The Right to Decide**. (*Note:* Check the virtual clock to see whether enough time has elapsed. You can use the fast-forward feature to advance the time by 2-minute intervals if the video is not yet available. Then click again on **Patient Care** and on **Nurse-Client Interactions** to refresh the screen.)

6. After considering data from the History and Physical and observing Goro Oishi's wife during the videos, you recognize a variety of factors influencing her perception of loss. For each of the following factors, describe the conditions affecting Mrs. Oishi's response to loss.

Nature of loss

Personal relationship

Culture

Spiritual belief

7. _____ In the event that Goro Oishi's son does not agree with Mrs. Oishi, her wishes will be deemed invalid. (True/False)

8. The grief being experienced by the Oishi family can best be described as:
   a. complicated grief.
   b. anticipatory grief.
   c. disenfranchised grief.
   d. disheartened grief.

 9. Goro Oishi has the following nursing diagnoses related to his numerous physical problems:
   • Impaired Gas Exchange
   • Risk for Aspiration
   • Risk for Impaired Skin Integrity
   • Impaired Bed Mobility

   What are the interrelationships among these nursing diagnoses? (*Hint:* See pages 248-249 in your textbook.)

 • Click on **Return to Room 505**.
• Click on **Leave the Floor** and then on **Restart the Program**.
• Sign in to work on the Skilled Nursing Floor, this time for Period of Care 3.
• From the Patient List, select Goro Oishi (Room 505).
• Click on **Get Report**; review the record and then click on **Go to Nurses' Station**.
• Click on **505** at the bottom of the screen.
• Review the Initial Observations.
• Click on **Patient Care** and then on **Nurse-Client Interactions**.
• Select and view the video titled **1500: Patient Decline**. (*Note:* Check the virtual clock to see whether enough time has elapsed. You can use the fast-forward feature to advance the time by 2-minute intervals if the video is not yet available. Then click again on **Patient Care** and on **Nurse-Client Interactions** to refresh the screen.)

10. Support of the grieving family is important at this time. In the video interaction, the nurse asks Mrs. Oishi to leave the bedside momentarily so that the nurse can speak with her. What purpose(s) does the nurse's action serve in supporting Mrs. Oishi? What other supportive intervention(s) could the nurse use?

11. Which of the following traditions are consistent with the Oishi family's religious practices? Select all that apply.

_____ The body should be placed on the floor, if possible, with the head facing north.

_____ The body should be buried as soon as possible after death.

_____ Burial is preferred to cremation.

_____ Prayers are often said while standing at the head of the deceased.

_____ Male family members are often asked to prepare the body.

_____ Gentle stroking of the arms and legs is considered a means to provide a relaxing transition to the afterlife.

12. According to the Grief Tasks Model, Mrs. Oishi would require a minimum of _____ to work through the grief tasks.
    a. 6 months
    b. 12 months
    c. 18 months
    d. 24 months

Exercise 3

Virtual Hospital Activity

30 minutes

- Sign in to work at Pacific View Regional Hospital on the Medical-Surgical Floor for Period of Care 1. (*Note:* If you are already in the virtual hospital from a previous exercise, click on **Leave the Floor** and then on **Restart the Program** to get to the sign-in window.)
- From the Patient List, select Harry George (Room 401).
- Click on **Get Report**; read the report and then click on **Go to Nurses' Station**.
- Click on **Chart** and then on **401**.
- Click on the **Nursing Admission** and then on **History and Physical**. Review the reports.

1. Harry George has experienced several different types of loss. Each type of loss is affected by the level of stress he has experienced. For each category below, identify the source of stress experienced by Harry George.

Situational

Maturational

Sociocultural

2. A focused assessment will help the nurse better understand the nature of stress affecting Harry George. For each of the assessment categories below, write two questions you would ask Harry George.

Perception of stressor

Adherence to healthy practices

3. Describe both the actual and perceived losses experienced by Harry George.

Actual

Perceived

4. For each of the following dimensions, describe a nursing intervention that would realistically promote hope for Harry George.

Cognitive dimension

Behavioral dimension

Contextual dimension

LESSON **9**

Vital Signs

Reading Assignment: Vital Signs (Chapter 29)
Fluid, Electrolyte, and Acid-Base Balance (Chapter 41,
pages 892 and 914)

Patients: Clarence Hughes, Medical-Surgical Floor, Room 404
Patricia Newman, Medical-Surgical Floor, Room 406

Objectives:

1. Recognize abnormal and normal vital signs.
2. Discuss techniques used to obtain accurate vital signs and physical assessment findings.
3. Describe interventions that can be implemented to manage vital sign abnormalities.

Exercise 1

Writing Activity

 30 minutes

1. What guidelines should be taken into consideration when incorporating vital signs into nursing practice?

2. The process by which the body regulates between heat lost and heat produced is known as

_____.

3. For each of the vital signs listed below, record the acceptable range for adults.

Temperature

Pulse

Respirations

Blood pressure

4. You are providing care for a 9-year-old patient. When assessing the heart rate, you know that which of the following findings is within normal limits?
   a. 60 to 90 beats per minute
   b. 90 to 140 beats per minute
   c. 75 to 100 beats per minute
   d. 100 to 120 beats per minute

5. You are taking the vital signs of a 10-year-old boy for a sports physical. During the assessment, you notice the child's heartbeat speeds up with inspiration and slows down with expiration. Which of the following actions should be taken *next*?
   a. Contact the physician.
   b. Obtain orders for an electrocardiogram (ECG).
   c. Instruct the child to hold his breath to further assess the phenomenon.
   d. Document the presence of a heart murmur.

6. Which part of the brain is responsible for control of body temperature?
   a. Hypothalamus
   b. Anterior pituitary gland
   c. Medulla
   d. Pons
   e. Cerebellum

7. The nurse is assessing a patient's respirations. The nurse notes that the patient's respiratory rate is 7 breaths per minute and that the depth of ventilation is depressed. Which of the following terms best describes the respiratory pattern being observed?
   a. Biot's respirations
   b. Cheyne-Stokes respirations
   c. Hypoventilation
   d. Kussmaul's respirations

8. A nurse has been advised to take a patient's temperature once daily. The nurse wants to take the temperature at the time when the patient would most likely have an elevation in reading. Based on your knowledge, you recognize the best time for the nurse to take the temperature would be:
   a. in the morning upon waking.
   b. in the middle of the day.
   c. in the early evening.
   d. just before bedtime.

9. A patient has an elevated temperature. Which of the following terms may be used to describe the patient's condition? Select all that apply.

_____ Afebrile

_____ Hyposphresia

_____ Febrile

_____ Pyretic

10. A heart rate less than 60 beats per minute is known as _____.

11. List at least six factors that may influence pulse rate.

12. Acceptable pulse oximetry ranges from _____ to _____. A value of less than _____ is considered hypoxemia. A value below _____ is acceptable for some conditions. (*Hint:* See page 476 in your textbook.)

13. A nurse is assessing a patient's pulse oxygen saturation readings. The nurse recognizes that which of the following factors may affect the results? Select all that apply.

_____ Patient motion

_____ Skin color

_____ Nail polish

_____ Fit of assessing probe

_____ Temperature at assessment site

14. _____ A potential site for pulse saturation level readings can be assessed for appropriateness by reviewing capillary refill. (True/False) (*Hint:* See pages 478-479 in your textbook.)

Exercise 2

Virtual Hospital Activity

45 minutes

- Sign in to work at Pacific View Regional Hospital on the Medical-Surgical Floor for Period of Care 2. (*Note:* If you are already in the virtual hospital from a previous exercise, click on **Leave the Floor** and then on **Restart the Program** to get to the sign-in window.)
- From the Patient List, select Clarence Hughes (Room 404).
- Click on **Get Report**.
- Click on **Go to Nurses' Station**.
- Click on **Chart** and then on **404**.
- Click on and review the **Physician's Orders**, **Physician's Notes**, **Admission Assessment**, and **History and Physical**.

1. Why has Clarence Hughes been admitted to the hospital?

2. Identify any significant factors in Clarence Hughes' medical history.

 - Click on **Return to Nurses' Station**.
- Click on **404** at the bottom of the screen.
- Review the Initial Observations.
- Click on **Take Vital Signs**.
- Click on and review the **Clinical Alerts**.

3. Record Clarence Hughes' vital signs below.

4. Clarence Hughes' heart rate is elevated. Which of the following is likely to be the underlying cause of the elevation?
   a. Fever
   b. Recent exercise
   c. Hypotension
   d. Decreased oxygenation

5. Based on his vital sign findings, what will be the best location for the nurse to assess Clarence Hughes' heart rate?
   a. Apical
   b. Brachial
   c. Radial
   d. Femoral

 6. If irregularities are noted in Clarence Hughes' heart rate, subsequent assessments should be counted for: (*Hint:* See page 473 in your textbook.)
   a. 10 seconds.
   b. 15 seconds.
   c. 30 seconds.
   d. 1 minute.

7. Develop a priority nursing diagnosis for Clarence Hughes that incorporates the abnormalities noted with his vital signs.

 • Click on **EPR** and then on **Login**.
   • Select **404** from the Patient drop-down menu and **Vital Signs** from the Category drop-down menu.
   • Review the vital signs recorded for Clarence Hughes since his admission.

8. When a nurse measures vital signs, technique may influence results. Which of the factors below could cause a false high value in Clarence Hughes' blood pressure. Select all that apply.

   _____ Loose-fitting cuff

   _____ Blood pressure cuff too wide

   _____ Inflation of blood pressure cuff too slow

   _____ Patient's arm above heart level

   _____ Blood pressure cuff deflated too quickly

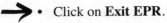 • Click on **Exit EPR**.
 • Click on **Patient Care** and then on **Physical Assessment**.

9. You are preparing to complete a physical examination for Clarence Hughes. As you review the body system categories listed below and on the next page (the yellow buttons on your screen), identify which subcategories (the green buttons) you believe are priorities for Clarence Hughes at this time? (*For example:* Under Head & Neck, would the Sensory area be a priority assessment?)

Head & Neck

Chest

Upper Extremities

Abdomen

Lower Extremities

• Complete a systems assessment by clicking on the body system categories (yellow buttons) and body system subcategories (green buttons).

10. Using the findings from your assessment of Clarence Hughes, match each of the following clinical manifestations with its probable cause.

Clinical Manifestation	Probable Cause
_____ Color in lower extremities pale	a. Anxious and agitated
_____ Attempt to improve ventilation	b. Tachypnea
_____ Pulmonary condition affecting oxygenation	c. Patient sitting up
_____ Reduced oxygen to brain	d. Altered peripheral circulation

 11. When Clarence Hughes' pulse oximetry reading is measured, it will normally take between

_____ and _____ seconds for the reading to appear. (*Hint:* See page 478 in your textbook.)

12. The nurse is preparing to obtain a pulse oximetry reading on Clarence Hughes. Which of the following are the two preferred locations?

_____ Tip of the nose

_____ Fingertip

_____ Lip

_____ Earlobe

• Click on **Chart**.
• Select the chart for Room **404**.
• Review the **Physician's Orders**. (*Note:* Click on **Return to Nurses' Station** and use the fast-forward feature to advance the clock to 1121. Click on **Chart** and then on **404**. Click on **Physician's Orders** to view the most recent orders.)

13. Explain the rationale for the arterial blood gas (ABG) orders.

Exercise 3

Virtual Hospital Activity

30 minutes

- Sign in to work at Pacific View Regional Hospital on the Medical-Surgical Floor for Period of Care 1. (*Note:* If you are already in the virtual hospital from a previous exercise, click on **Leave the Floor** and then on **Restart the Program** to get to the sign-in window.)
- From the Patient List, select Patricia Newman (Room 406).
- Click on **Get Report**.
- Click on **Go to Nurses' Station**.
- Click on **Chart** and then on **406**.
- Click on and then review the **Nursing Admission** and **History and Physical**.

1. Why has Patricia Newman been admitted to the hospital?

2. What factors in Patricia Newman's health history may be associated with her emphysema and hypertension?

3. While assessing Patricia Newman, the nurse hears coarse crackles throughout the lung fields. Below, identify the characteristics of crackles. Select all that apply. (*Hint:* See Table 30-22 in your textbook.)

_____ Heard over anterior lateral lung field

_____ Best heard in dependent lobes

_____ Primarily heard over trachea and bronchi

_____ Caused by high-velocity air flow

_____ Result of inflamed pleura

_____ Result of sudden reinflation of alveoli

_____ High-pitched, fine, and short sound

_____ Dry grating sound

_____ Low-pitched rumbling sound

• Click on **Return to Nurses' Station**.
- Click on **406** to go to Patricia Newman's room.
- Review the Initial Observations.
- Click on **Take Vital Signs** and review.

4. Record the vital signs for Patricia Newman below.

5. Which of Patricia Newman's vital signs are abnormal?

 • Click on **Patient Care** and then on **Nurse-Client Interactions**.
- Select and view the video titled **0730: Prioritizing Interventions**. (*Note:* Check the virtual clock to see whether enough time has elapsed. You can use the fast-forward feature to advance the time by 2-minute intervals if the video is not yet available. Then click again on **Patient Care** and on **Nurse-Client Interactions** to refresh the screen.)
- After viewing the video, click on **Physical Assessment**.
- Complete a focused assessment by clicking on **Chest** (yellow buttons) and then on the available body system subcategories (green buttons).

6. During the nurse-client interaction, the nurse indicates that she plans to administer a prescribed antipyretic medication for Patricia Newman's fever. What additional interventions can be implemented to manage the febrile patient?

7. Match the blood pressure types listed below with the corresponding auscultatory sound. (*Note:* Not all of the auscultatory sounds will be used.)

Blood Pressure Type	Auscultatory Sound
_____ Systolic	a. First Korotkoff sound
_____ Diastolic	b. Second Korotkoff sound
	c. Third Korotkoff sound
	d. Fourth Korotkoff sound
	e. Fifth Korotkoff sound

8. Patricia Newman may exhibit an auscultatory gap during her assessment. What factor in her health history/current diagnosis will increase the incidence for the development of this phenomenon?
   a. Elevated temperature
   b. Increased heart rate
   c. Elevated blood pressure
   d. Reduced lung capability
   e. Increased respirations

9. What is an auscultatory gap, and between which Korotkoff sounds does it typically occur?

10. What actions can you take to avoid having this happen?

Medication Administration

 Reading Assignment: Medication Administration (Chapter 31)

Patients: Piya Jordan, Medical-Surgical Floor, Room 403
Kathryn Doyle, Skilled Nursing Floor, Room 503

Objectives:

1. Discuss the rationale for the medications ordered for two patients.
2. Explain the six rights of medication administration.
3. Perform medication dosage calculations.
4. Identify potential sources of medication errors.
5. Describe the steps required for medication administration.

Exercise 1

Writing Activity

30 minutes

1. The _____ name of a medication is an exact description of its composition and molecular structure.

2. The trade name, brand name, or _____ name is the official name under which a manufacturer markets a medication.

3. After taking a prescribed medication, a patient reports feeling very tired. The nurse caring for the patient consults a drug handbook and determines that the medication is not associated with drowsiness. What term is used to refer to this type of patient reaction?
   a. Side effect
   b. Adverse effect
   c. Toxic effect
   d. Idiosyncratic reaction
   e. Allergic reaction

4. Below are abbreviations commonly associated with medication administration. Match each abbreviation with its correct meaning.

Abbreviation	Meaning
_____ ad lib	a. Give immediately
_____ AC	b. As desired
_____ qAM	c. After meals
_____ STAT	d. Every morning
_____ PC	e. Before meals
_____ prn	f. Whenever there is a need

5. The physician has ordered laboratory studies to evaluate the peak and trough of a medication. Which of the following statements concerning these terms is correct? Select all that apply.

   _____ Peak refers to the time it takes for a medication to produce a response after it is administered.

   _____ Peak refers to the time it takes for a medication to reach its highest effective concentration.

   _____ Trough refers to the length of time of the therapeutic response produced by a medication.

   _____ Trough refers to the smallest serum concentration of medication present before the next scheduled dosage.

   _____ Trough refers to the amount of medication needed to produce a therapeutic response.

6. When two medications have a(n) _____, their combined effect is greater than the effect of the medications given separately.

7. _____ Medications intended for sublingual administration may not have the desired effect if swallowed. (True/False)

8. Which of the following statements describe activities for correctly following the six rights of medication administration? Select all that apply.

   _____ Compare the MAR with the physician's written order for the name of a medication.

   _____ Review the patient record for allergies.

   _____ Review the supply cart for available sizes of syringes.

   _____ Check the MAR against the physician's written order for the route of administration.

   _____ Compare the physician's written order for a medication with the times selected on the MAR for scheduled administration.

9. Which of the following sites is preferred for administering an intramuscular (IM) injection to an adult?
   a. Vastus lateralis
   b. Ventrogluteal
   c. Deltoid
   d. Dorsogluteal

10. What is the Z-track method? What is the benefit of using this method?

11. Below, identify the characteristics of the Z-track method. Select all that apply.

   _____ Technique for administering intramuscular (IM) injections

   _____ Minimizes local skin irritation

   _____ Allows medication to escape from the muscle tissue

   _____ Seals medication in muscle tissue

   _____ Needle remains inserted for 30 seconds to allow for even dispersal of medication

12. List the six rights of medication administration.

13. Identify the four steps involved in the process for medication reconciliation.

Exercise 2

  Virtual Hospital Activity

 15 minutes

- Sign in to work at Pacific View Regional Hospital on the Medical-Surgical Floor for Period of Care 1. (*Note:* If you are already in the virtual hospital from a previous exercise, click on **Leave the Floor** and then on **Restart the Program** to get to the sign-in window.)
- From the Patient List, select Piya Jordan (Room 403).
- Click on **Get Report**.
- Click on **Go to Nurses' Station**.
- Click on **Chart** and select the chart for Room **403**.
- Click on and review the **History and Physical**.
- Click on and review the **Physician's Orders** for Tuesday and Wednesday mornings.
- Click on **Return to Nurse's Station** and then click on the **Drug** icon in the lower left-hand corner of the screen.

1. Piya Jordan has orders for a number of medications postoperatively. Match each medication listed below with the rationale for its administration.

Medication	Rationale
_____ Digoxin 0.125 mg IV	a. Reduce fever
_____ Famotidine 20 mg IV	b. Reduce gastric acid secretion
_____ Cefotetan 2 g IV	c. Slow the heart rate of atrial fibrillation
_____ Acetaminophen 650 mg per rectum q6h	d. Prevent postoperative wound infection

- Click on **Return to Nurses' Station**.
- Click on the **Medication Room** at the bottom of your screen.
- Click on **MAR** and then on tab **403**.
- Review the MAR for drugs due to be given Wednesday between 0730 and 0815.
- Click on **Return to Medication Room**.
- Based on your review of the MAR, access the storage areas of the Medication Room to obtain the needed medications for administration.
- For each area you access, select the medication you plan to administer and then click on **Put Medication on Tray**. When finished with a storage area, click on **Close Drawer** or **Close Bin**.
- Click on **View Medication Room**.
- Now click on **Preparation** and choose the correct medication to administer.
- Click on **Prepare** and then click on **Next**. Choose the correct patient to administer this medication to.
- Complete the Preparation Wizard by providing any information requested. When the Wizard stops asking for information, click on **Finish**.
- You can click on **Review Your Medications** and then on **Return to Medication Room** when ready.

2. _____ mL of digoxin should have been prepared for Piya Jordan.

3. Which of the following medications did you prepare for this time period? Select all that apply.

_____ Enoxaparin 40 mg

_____ 20 mEq potassium chloride in 250 mL normal saline

_____ Digoxin 0.125 mg

_____ Morphine sulfate 2.5 mg per mL

_____ Cefotetan 1 g

→ • Click on **Nurses' Station** at the bottom of the screen.
  • Click on **403** at the bottom of the screen.

4. What should be assessed before the ordered dose of digoxin is administered to Piya Jordan? (*Hint:* Refer to the Drug Guide.)
   a. Blood pressure and IV infusion
   b. Apical heart and IV infusion
   c. Potassium level and blood pressure
   d. Patient's level of discomfort and range of motion in knees

5. Digoxin must be given over a(n) _____-minute period of time.

6. Before you administer the digoxin, what should be included in the assessment of the IV infusion?

7. Knowledge of potential signs of toxicity are important to providing quality care. What manifestations could indicate the presence of digoxin toxicity in Piya Jordan? Select all that apply.

_____ Increased nausea

_____ Visual changes

_____ Headache

_____ Nasal stuffiness

_____ Irritability

• Perform any necessary assessments and review any pertinent information before administering the medications that you prepared.

  • After you have collected the appropriate assessment data and when you are ready for administration, click on **Patient Care** and then on **Medication Administration**.

  • Verify that the correct patient and medication(s) appear in the left-hand window.

  • Click the down arrow next to Select. From the drop-down menu, select **Administer** and complete the Administration Wizard by providing any information requested. When the Wizard stops asking for information, click on **Administer to Patient**. Specify **Yes** when asked whether this administration should be recorded in the MAR.

  • Click on **Finish**.

  8. _____ IV administration of digoxin creates a greater risk to the patient than IV administration of potassium chloride. (True/False)

Exercise 3

 ### Virtual Hospital Activity

 30 minutes

  • Sign in to work at Pacific View Regional Hospital on the Medical-Surgical Floor for Period of Care 2. (*Note:* If you are already in the virtual hospital from a previous exercise, click on **Leave the Floor** and then on **Restart the Program** to get to the sign-in window.)

  • From the Patient List, select Piya Jordan (Room 403)

  • Click on **Get Report** and then on **Go to Nurses' Station**.

  • Click on **Chart** and then on **403**.

  • Click on and then review the **History and Physical**, **Nurse's Notes**, and **Physician's Orders**.

  1. The physician has ordered ondansetron 4 mg IV q6h prn for nausea. Which of the following statements is true about a prn order?
     a. It calls for a single dose of a medication to be given only once.
     b. It is a type of order that requires the medication be given at a specific time.
     c. It is an order prescribed for a time when a patient requires it.
     d. It is the only type of order canceled when a patient goes to surgery.

  2. The physician has ordered enoxaparin 40 mg subQ. The administration of this medication

     will require a(n) _____-gauge needle.

  3. When preparing to administer the enoxaparin, you may use a(n) _____- to _____-mL syringe.

  4. Which of the following sites is the best location for administering enoxaparin to Piya Jordan?
     a. Deltoid
     b. Abdomen
     c. Thigh
     d. Buttocks

5. The angle range for administering a subcutaneous injection is 45 to 90 degrees. What factors will be used to determine the correct angle placement for administering the subcutaneous injection to Piya Jordan?

 • Click on **Return to Nurses' Station**.
 • Click on **403** at the bottom of the screen.
 • Review the Initial Observations.
 • Click on **Patient Care** and then on **Nurse-Client Interactions**.
 • Select and view the video titled **1115: Interventions—Nausea, Blood**. (*Note:* Check the virtual clock to see whether enough time has elapsed. You can use the fast-forward feature to advance the time by 2-minute intervals if the video is not yet available. Then click again on **Patient Care** and on **Nurse-Client Interactions** to refresh the screen.)
 • After viewing the video, click on **Take Vital Signs**.
 • Click on **MAR** and then on tab **403**.

6. During the video interaction, the nurse communicates plans to administer Tylenol to Piya Jordan. Has this medication been ordered by the physician? Are any additional actions needed before this medication can be administered?

7. Piya Jordan has complained of nausea. _____ has been prescribed to manage the nausea.

 • Click on **Return to Room 403**.
 • Click on **Medication Room** at the bottom of your screen.
 • Click on **Unit Dosage** and then on the drawer for Room **403**.
 • Select the antiemetic. Place the medication on the tray.
 • Click on **Close Drawer** and then click on **Review Your Medications**.
 • Click on **View Medication Room** and then on **Preparation**.

8. Ondansetron is available in a strength of _____ mg/mL.

9. The available vial of ondansetron contains _____ mL.

10. The physician has ordered a dosage of _____ mg of ondansetron to be administered every 6 hours prn as needed for nausea.

11. _____ It is necessary to dilute ondansetron with D_5W before administering the medication by way of IV push. (True/False)

12. Listed below are steps describing the proper technique for administering an IV push medication. Match the columns to show correct order of these steps.

Steps for Administering IV Push	Order
_____ Clean off injection port with antiseptic swab	a. 1
_____ Recheck fluid infusion rate	b. 2
_____ Perform hand hygiene and apply gloves	c. 3
_____ Select injection port of IV tubing closest to patient	d. 4
_____ Check patient's identification by looking at identification bracelet and asking the patient his or her name	e. 5
	f. 6
_____ Occlude IV line and check for blood return	
	g. 7
_____ Withdraw syringe from port	
	h. 8
_____ Connect syringe to IV line	
	i. 9
_____ Dispose of uncapped needles and syringe and perform hand hygiene	
	j. 10
_____ Release tubing and inject medication within time recommended	

13. Headache, chest pain, and difficulty breathing can be side effects of ondansetron. If Piya Jordan develops any of these, what would you do?

Exercise 4

  Virtual Hospital Activity

 15 minutes

- Sign in to work at Pacific View Regional Hospital on the Skilled Nursing Floor for Period of Care 2. (*Note:* If you are already in the virtual hospital from a previous exercise, click on **Leave the Floor** and then on **Restart the Program** to get to the sign-in window.)
- From the Patient List, select Kathryn Doyle (Room 503).
- Click on **Get Report**; review the report and then click on **Go to Nurses' Station**.
- Click on **Chart** and then on **503**.
- Click on and then review the **History and Physical**, **Nurse's Notes**, and **Physician's Orders**.

1. In what manner can Kathryn Doyle's issues with dehydration be managed or improved during the administration of oral medications?

2. Match each of the medications ordered for Kathryn Doyle with its appropriate purpose. (*Hint:* Refer to the Drug Guide as needed.)

Medication	Purpose
_____ Calcium citrate	a. Treatment for anemia
_____ Ferrous sulfate	b. Prevention of infection
_____ Docusate sodium	c. Prevention of constipation
_____ Ibuprofen	d. Treatment for osteoporosis
	e. Improvement of appetite
	f. Relief of pain in left hip

➡ - Click on **Return to Nurses' Station**.
- Click on **Medication Room**.

3. What patient data should be checked before beginning to remove medications from the dispensing system? Select all that apply.

_____ Fluid intake for last 8 hours

_____ Vital signs at 0700

_____ Medication Administration Record

_____ Activity order

_____ Allergy record

4. Two medications prescribed for Kathryn Doyle can cause constipation. Which drugs are they?
   a. Ferrous sulfate and docusate sodium
   b. Calcium citrate and ibuprofen
   c. Ibuprofen and ferrous sulfate
   d. Ferrous sulfate and calcium citrate

5. Kathryn Doyle has documented issues with dehydration. If she asks you to crush her medications and mix them with applesauce, what actions are indicated?

6. Discuss actions that must be taken when preparing to crush medications. Discuss the associated rationale.

7. Which of the following side effects is of the most concern when administering ibuprofen?
   a. Gastrointestinal distress
   b. Headache
   c. Black stools
   d. Urinary frequency

8. When planning Kathryn Doyle's care, you must remember that medications are to be

   administered within _____ minutes of their ordered time.

LESSON 11

Activity and Mobility

 Reading Assignment: Managing Patient Care (Chapter 21, pages 281-283)
Activity and Exercise (Chapter 38)
Mobility and Immobility (Chapter 47)

Patient: Kathryn Doyle, Skilled Nursing Floor, Room 503

Objectives:

1. Identify changes in physiologic function associated with immobility.
2. Formulate appropriate nursing diagnoses for the patient with immobility.
3. Review assistive devices for the patient with impaired mobility.
4. Discuss interventions to manage the patient with impaired mobility.

Exercise 1

 Writing Activity

20 minutes

1. What chronic disorders are affected by activity and exercise?

2. A nurse is teaching a patient to use a cane. How far ahead of the patient's feet should the cane be placed?
   a. No distance, keep the cane even with the feet
   b. 3 to 5 inches
   c. 6 to 10 inches
   d. At least 12 inches

3. A patient reports being confused about the differences between isometric and isotonic exercise. Which of the following statements made by the nurse is correct?
   a. "Isotonic exercises are best for those who are unable to tolerate much activity."
   b. "Isotonic exercises do not have an impact on muscle mass or tone."
   c. "Isometric exercises are beneficial for hospitalized individuals."
   d. "Isometric exercises will do little to increase endurance."

4. A physician has recommended that a patient engage in resistive isometric exercises. Which of the following would be appropriate for this type of activity?
   a. Walking
   b. Stationary bicycling
   c. Push-ups
   d. Quadriceps set exercise

5. A nurse is preparing a patient to perform range-of-motion (ROM) exercises. The nurse correctly recognizes that the range of movement for the forearm is:
   a. 60 degrees.
   b. 70 to 90 degrees.
   c. 150 degrees.
   d. 320 degrees.

6. For what symptoms should a nurse monitor a patient when performing ROM exercises?

7. Unless contraindicated by a medical condition, it is recommended that an adult drink at

   least _____ to _____ mL of noncaffeinated fluids daily to maintain normal mucociliary clearance.

8. A patient with alterations in neurologic function reports being unable to establish spatial

   positioning of the body. The patient is demonstrating problems with _____.

9. To determine metabolic functioning, _____ measurements may be assessed.

10. Calcium intake is needed to promote strong bones and teeth. Which of the following foods are rich in calcium? Select all that apply.

_____ Yogurt

_____ Oranges

_____ Cheese

_____ Kale

_____ Bananas

11. A patient inquires about kyphosis. Which of the following statements would be appropriate to include in the discussion? Select all that apply.

_____ "Kyphosis involves an abnormal curvature of the cervical spine."

_____ "Kyphosis may have congenital causes."

_____ "Treatments for kyphosis may include vitamin D and calcium supplements."

_____ "The use of a bed board may be used in the management of kyphosis."

_____ "Kyphosis is the result of a curvature in the thoracic spine."

12. _____ Footdrop can be corrected with exercises. (True/False)

Exercise 2

Virtual Hospital Activity

30 minutes

- Sign in to work at Pacific View Regional Hospital on the Skilled Nursing Floor for Period of Care 2. (*Note:* If you are already in the virtual hospital from a previous exercise, click on **Leave the Floor** and then on **Restart the Program** to get to the sign-in window.)
- From the Patient List, select Kathryn Doyle (Room 503).
- Click on **Get Report**; read the report and then click on **Go to Nurses' Station**.
- Click on **Chart** and then on **503**.
- Click on and then review the **Nursing Admission**, **Nurse's Notes**, **Physician's Orders**, and **History and Physical**.

1. What is Kathryn Doyle's primary diagnosis?

2. What other chronic health problems are in Kathryn Doyle's medical history?

3. Which of the following statements concerning osteoporosis is correct? Select all that apply.

_____ "Only women can get osteoporosis."

_____ "By the year 2020, one in two Americans over the age of 50 will be at risk for an osteoporosis-related fracture."

_____ "The goal of the patient with osteoporosis is to maintain independence with activities of daily living (ADLs)."

_____ "Immobility is a risk factor for the development of osteoporosis."

_____ "Small-framed individuals are at a lower risk for developing osteoporosis."

4. _____ Kathryn Doyle can begin to develop contractures after only 8 hours of immobility. (True/False)

5. Which of the following orders reflect the physician's plan concerning Kathryn Doyle's activity? Select all that apply.

_____ Ambulate prn

_____ Physical therapy to direct rehabilitation

_____ Ambulate at least four times daily

_____ May use bed pan if desired

_____ Activity as tolerated

6. When the nurse is planning care for Kathryn Doyle, which of the following tasks may be delegated to nursing assistive personnel? Select all that apply. (*Hint:* See pages 281-283 in your textbook.)

_____ Assess Kathryn Doyle's exercise tolerance after ambulation

_____ Evaluate joint limitation with movement

_____ Obtain vital signs before exercise

_____ Obtain vital signs after exercise

_____ Assist patient with ambulation

7. The Nurse's Notes for Wednesday morning state that Kathryn Doyle refused to ambulate to the dining room for breakfast and to work with physical therapy. What impact can immobility have on bone health?

8. _____ Based on data provided, there are physiologic factors preventing Kathryn Doyle from ambulating to the dining room. (True/False)

9. _____ Kathryn Doyle's risk for orthostatic hypotension is increased by her immobility. (True/False)

10. What consultations have been ordered by the physician to assist Kathryn Doyle in managing her physiologic and psychologic problems?

11. Which of the following assistive devices are appropriate for Kathryn Doyle's use? Select all that apply.

    _____ Trapeze bar

    _____ Crutches

    _____ Walker

    _____ Cane

    _____ Wheel chair

→ • Click on **Return to Nurses' Station**.
   • Click on **EPR** and then on **Login**.
   • Select **503** from the Patient drop-down menu and **Nutrition** from the Category drop-down menu. Review the findings.
   • Select **Intake and Output** from the Category drop-down menu and then review the findings.

Kathryn Doyle's history reveals a poor appetite. She has not consumed an entire meal since her admission. She is at risk for a negative nitrogen balance unless she becomes more active and mobile. Fill in the blanks in the statements below.

12. Kathryn Doyle's immobilization causes muscle _____, which leads to negative nitrogen balance.

13. Kathryn Doyle's reported weight loss is a result of _____ catabolism.

• Click on **Exit EPR**.
• Click on **503** at the bottom of the screen.
• Click on **Patient Care** and then on **Physical Assessment**.
• Complete a full body assessment by clicking on the body system categories (yellow buttons) and subcategories (green buttons).

14. What assessments may be done to check Kathryn Doyle for a deep vein thrombosis?

15. Review any abnormal findings discovered during your assessment of the respiratory system. How do these findings relate to Kathryn Doyle's immobility?

16. What interventions can be implemented to assist in managing the concerns addressed in the preceding question?

Oxygenation

 Reading Assignment: Oxygenation (Chapter 40)

Patients: Jacquline Catanazaro, Medical-Surgical Floor, Room 402
Patricia Newman, Medical-Surgical Floor, Room 406

Objectives:

1. Describe cardiac output, stroke volume, preload, and afterload.
2. Review the impact of a patient's level of health, age, lifestyle, and environment on oxygenation.
3. Review the assessment and nursing care for a patient with impaired oxygenation.

Exercise 1

 Writing Activity

15 minutes

1. Match each of the following terms associated with myocardial blood flow with its correct definition.

Term	Definition
_____ Cardiac output	a. The end-diastolic volume
_____ Stroke volume	b. The volume of blood ejected from the ventricles during systole
_____ Preload	c. The resistance to left ventricular ejection
_____ Afterload	d. The volume of blood ejected from the left ventricle each minute

2. The term _____ is used to refer to inadequate tissue oxygenation at the cellular level.

3. The process of adding water to a gas is known as _____.

4. While reviewing a patient's medical record, a nurse notes a history of atelectasis. Based on your understanding, you recognize that this condition results when there is:
   a. an imbalance between myocardial oxygen demands and the available supply.
   b. an excessive ventilation of the alveoli.
   c. a collapse of the alveoli.
   d. a lack of available circulating hemoglobin.

5. Which of the following risk factors are modifiable in regard to the development of cardiovascular disease? Select all that apply.

   _____ Age

   _____ Smoking

   _____ Gender

   _____ Heredity

   _____ Weight

   _____ Lack of exercise

6. While auscultating the patient's lung fields, the nurse notes the presence of a high-pitched musical sound. Which of the following sounds has the nurse likely heard?
   a. Rales
   b. Wheezes
   c. Rhonchi
   d. Crackles

7. The nurse is collecting information related to the patient's health history. The patient reports having undergone a test a few years ago for which the patient wore a portable monitor for 24 hours to "check [his] heart." The patient cannot recall the name of the test. Based on your knowledge, you recognize that the patient is most likely referring to which of the following?
   a. Scintigraphy
   b. ECG exercise stress test
   c. Thallium stress test
   d. Holter monitor

8. _____ Forgetfulness and irritability are often the first signs of respiratory problems. (True/False)

9. _____ The majority of tuberculosis (TB) cases occur in racial and ethnic minorities. (True/False)

Exercise 2

Virtual Hospital Activity

45 minutes

- Sign in to work at Pacific View Regional Hospital on the Medical-Surgical Floor for Period of Care 1. (*Note:* If you are already in the virtual hospital from a previous exercise, click on **Leave the Floor** and then on **Restart the Program** to get to the sign-in window).
- From the Patient List, select Patricia Newman (Room 406).
- Click on **Get Report** and then on **Go to Nurses' Station**.
- Click on **Chart** and then on **406**.
- Click on and review the **Nursing Admission**, **Physician's Notes**, **History and Physical**, and **Laboratory Reports**.

1. What is Patricia Newman's admitting diagnosis?

2. What are the significant findings in Patricia Newman's medical history?

3. Which of the following physiologic changes in oxygenation have resulted from Patricia Newman's admitting diagnosis?

_____ Impaired ventilatory movement

_____ Decreased hemoglobin level

_____ Decreased diffusion of oxygen from the alveoli to the blood

_____ Instability of tissues to extract oxygen from the blood

_____ Obstruction of airways with mucus

4. Patricia Newman has a long-standing history of emphysema. For each of the following physiologic changes associated with emphysema, provide a rationale that explains the change.

Increased work of breathing

Fatigue

Dyspnea on exertion

Elevated $PaCO_2$

5. Which of the following factors in Patricia Newman's medical history place her at an increased risk for the development of pneumonia? Select all that apply.

_____ Smoking

_____ Hypertension

_____ Osteoporosis

_____ Social isolation

_____ Hysterectomy

_____ Emphysema

6. When planning care for Patricia Newman, an understanding of emphysema is important. Which of the following statements regarding the disorder are correct? Select all that apply.

_____ Emphysema affects both men and women.

_____ Symptoms typically begin to manifest when patients are in their mid- to late 30s.

_____ The disorder is characterized by changes in the alveolar walls and capillaries.

_____ Disability often results in patients diagnosed with emphysema between the ages of 50 and 60 years.

_____ Heredity may play a role in the development of emphysema.

7. How will the physician determine which medication is best to treat Patricia Newman's pneumonia?

8. The physician has ordered oxygen at 2 L per nasal cannula. Which of the following statements about this method of delivery is correct?
   a. Oxygen per nasal cannula is drying to mucous membranes.
   b. The use of the nasal cannula interferes with eating and talking.
   c. The use of the nasal cannula is an expensive means of oxygen delivery.
   d. The nasal cannula is an effective way to provide humidified oxygen.

- Click on **Return to Nurses' Station**.
- Click on **406** at the bottom of the screen.
- Review the Initial Observations.
- Click on **Take Vital Signs** and review.
- Click on **Patient Care** and then on **Physical Assessment**.
- Review the assessments for **Head & Neck**, **Chest**, and **Back & Spine**.

9. What are Patricia Newman's vital signs?

10. Patricia Newman's oxygen saturation is _____.

11. The physician has ordered oxygen therapy via nasal cannula at 2 L. What are the implications of increasing the oxygen to Patricia Newman?

12. Hypoventilation in the patient with chronic obstructive pulmonary disease (COPD) can result in which of the following conditions?
   a. Metabolic acidosis
   b. Metabolic alkalosis
   c. Respiratory acidosis
   d. Respiratory alkalosis

13. What findings on the respiratory assessment provide support for the admitting diagnosis?

14. _____ Patricia Newman's use of accessory muscles for breathing will ultimately increase her pulmonary capacity. (True/False)

15. _____ The stimulus for Patricia Newman to breathe is a lack of available oxygen. (True/False)

16. What nursing interventions can be implemented to improve airway clearance?

17. Patricia Newman has tachycardia. Which of the following factors is a causative factor for this? Select all that apply.

   _____ Tobacco use

   _____ Estrogen patch use

   _____ Pain

   _____ Hypoxia

   _____ Hypertension

18. Patricia Newman's assessment reveals the following physical findings: $PaCO_2$ 47; dyspnea on exertion; naps frequently; abnormal rate and depth of breathing. Based on these findings, what is the most appropriate nursing diagnosis?
   a. Ineffective Breathing Pattern
   b. Ineffective Tissue Perfusion
   c. Impaired Gas Exchange
   d. Ineffective Airway Clearance

Exercise 3

Virtual Hospital Activity

30 minutes

- Sign in to work at Pacific View Regional Hospital on the Medical-Surgical Floor for Period of Care 1. (*Note:* If you are already in the virtual hospital from a previous exercise, click on **Leave the Floor** and then on **Restart the Program** to get to the sign-in window.)
- From the Patient List, select Jacquline Catanazaro (Room 402).
- Click on **Get Report**.
- Click on **Go to Nurses' Station**.
- Click on **Chart** and select the chart for Room **402**.
- Click on and review the **Nursing Admission** and **History and Physical**.

1. Why has Jacquline Catanazaro been admitted to the hospital?

2. Which of the following risk factors for the development of respiratory illness are present for Jacquline Catanazaro? Select all that apply.

_____ Age

_____ History of travel

_____ Occupational exposures

_____ Smoking

_____ Family history

_____ Inactivity

3. At times, Jacquline Catanazaro reportedly becomes very anxious from her mental illness. Which of the following best describes the influence anxiety has on the patient's oxygenation status?
   a. Causes hypoventilation
   b. Increases the body's metabolic rate and oxygen demand
   c. Reduces the diffusion of oxygen across the alveolar membrane
   d. Creates a sense of breathlessness from CO_2 retention

4. The physician ordered STAT nebulization for Jacquline Catanazaro using albuterol. Nebulization will most likely improve her ability to breathe by what mechanism(s)? Select all that apply. (*Hint:* Click on the **Drug** icon to review albuterol.)

_____ Decreasing the volume of sputum to expectorate

_____ Cooling inhaled air

_____ Relieving bronchospasm

_____ Enhancing mucociliary clearance

_____ Reducing the patient's peak flow rate

→ • Click on **Return to Nurses' Station**.
   • Click on **402** at the bottom of the screen.
   • Review the Initial Observations.
   • Click on **Patient Care** and then on **Nurse-Client Interactions**.
   • Select and view the video titled **0730: Intervention—Airway**. (*Note:* Check the virtual clock to see whether enough time has elapsed. You can use the fast-forward feature to advance the time by 2-minute intervals if the video is not yet available. Then click again on **Patient Care** and on **Nurse-Client Interactions** to refresh the screen.)
   • Next, click on **Physical Assessment** and conduct a focused assessment based on Jacquline Catanazaro's current condition.

5. Identify the abnormalities in Jacquline Catanazaro's respiratory assessment.

6. Match each of Jacquline Catanazaro's physical findings with the corresponding physiologic change.

Physical Finding	Physiologic Change
_____ Hyperresonance to percussion	a. Increased airway resistance
_____ Substernal retraction	b. High-velocity airflow
_____ Tachypnea	c. Air-filled lungs
_____ Wheezes bilaterally	d. Decreased oxygen levels trigger increased respiratory rate
_____ Peak flow meter shows value of 200	e. Increased work of breathing

7. Jacquline Catanazaro's skin is noted as being moist and clammy. What significance does this have in relation to her respiratory status?

8. During the respiratory crisis being experienced by Jacquline Catanazaro, what is the priority nursing diagnosis?
   a. Activity Intolerance
   b. Anxiety
   c. Impaired Gas Exchange
   d. Ineffective Health Maintenance

9. What are Jacquline Catanazaro's vital signs?

10. Jacquline Catanazaro is experiencing significant respiratory distress. What has been ordered to manage the attack?

11. Jacquline Catanazaro's pulse oximeter reading is _____%.

12. The pulse oximeter reading is the:
    a. blood's hemoglobin level.
    b. oxygen saturation of hemoglobin in the blood.
    c. the body's level of $PaCO_2$.
    d. the body's acid-base balance.

13. The following medications have been prescribed to manage Jacquline Catanazaro's breathing difficulties. Match the prescribed medication with the correct mode of action.

Medication	Mode of Action
_____ Beclomethasone	a. Relief of bronchospasms
_____ Albuterol	b. Reduction of bronchial inflammation
_____ Ipratropium bromide	c. Control of secretions

• Click on **Leave the Floor**.
- From the Floor Menu, select **Restart the Program**.
- Sign in to work at Pacific View Regional Hospital on the Medical-Surgical Floor for Period of Care 1.
- From the Patient List, select Jacquline Catanazaro (Room 402).
- Click on **Go to Nurses' Station**.
- Click on **Chart** and select the chart for Room **402**.
- Click on and review the **Physician's Notes** and the **Physician's Orders**.

14. The physician's notes for 0800 and 1000 show two sets of arterial blood gas (ABG) values:

    0800: pH 7.38, PaO_2 80, $PaCO_2$ 50, HCO_3 26, O_2 sat 85%

    1000: pH 7.40, PaO_2 92, $PaCO_2$ 40, HCO_3 23, O_2 sat 99%

    What is the reason for the change in Jacquline Catanazaro's ABG values?

15. Jacquline Catanazaro has a productive cough with frothy secretions. Why is tracheal suctioning inadvisable?

LESSON 13

Fluid, Electrolyte, and Acid-Base Balance

 Reading Assignment: Oxygenation (Chapter 40)
Fluid, Electrolyte, and Acid-Base Balance (Chapter 41)
Care of Surgical Patients (Chapter 50)

Patients: Piya Jordan, Medical-Surgical Floor, Room 403
Patricia Newman, Medical-Surgical Floor, Room 406

Objectives:

1. Identify disturbances in fluid and electrolyte balances in two patients.
2. Describe variables that affect fluid and electrolyte balance.
3. Describe the factors to include in the assessment of a peripheral intravenous (PIV) site.
4. Calculate an intravenous (IV) flow rate.

Exercise 1

 Writing Activity

15 minutes

1. Body fluids are divided between two distinct compartments. The fluids within the cells are

known as _____. Fluids outside of the cells are known as

_____.

2. Identify the three processes at play in fluid homeostasis.

3. A nurse is reviewing the results of a patient's electrolyte panel. The documentation indicates the patient's potassium level is 5.2 mEq/L, a level that is indicative of:
   a. hypopotassium.
   b. hyperkalemia.
   c. hypernatremia.
   d. hypercalcemia.

4. A patient is being treated for hypocalcemia. Based on your knowledge, which of the following disorders might contribute to this disorder?
   a. Pancreatitis
   b. Excess aldosterone secretion
   c. Psychogenic polydipsia
   d. Diabetes insipidus

5. _____ The most effective means by which to monitor acid-base balance is by examination of arterial blood gas (ABG) values. (True/False)

6. _____ When the nurse is providing fluid maintenance for an adult, the use of a peripheral 18-gauge cannula is appropriate. (True/False)

7. Which of the following patient populations are at increased risk for developing fluid, electrolyte, and acid-base imbalances? Select all that apply.

   _____ Older adults

   _____ Infants

   _____ Males

   _____ Patients with burn injuries

   _____ Patients using oral contraceptives

8. A patient is taking prescribed steroids. Which of the following complications should the nurse be aware of related to the use of this medication?
   a. Metabolic alkalosis
   b. Hypokalemia
   c. Nephrotoxicity
   d. Metabolic acidosis

9. When preparing for a blood transfusion, it is important to prime the tubing with _____ to prevent hemolysis of red blood cells.
   a. 5% dextrose
   b. Lactated Ringer's
   c. 0.9% sodium chloride (normal saline)
   d. 10% dextrose

Exercise 2

Virtual Hospital Activity

30 minutes

- Sign in to work at Pacific View Regional Hospital on the Medical-Surgical Floor for Period of Care 1. (*Note:* If you are already in the virtual hospital from a previous exercise, click on **Leave the Floor** and then on **Restart the Program** to get to the sign-in window.
- From the Patient List, select Piya Jordan (Room 403).
- Click on **Get Report**; read the report and then click on **Go to Nurses' Station**.
- Click on **Chart** and then on **403**.
- Click on and review the **Nursing Admission**.

1. Identify three factors in Piya Jordan's Nursing Admission data that indicate a risk for fluid and electrolyte imbalances even before surgery.

2. Consider the data you received from the change-of-shift report. From the following list, identify the risks Piya Jordan has for fluid and electrolyte imbalance during the post-operative period. Select all that apply.

_____ Taking digoxin at home

_____ Nasogastric (NG) tube draining a moderate amount of brown fluid

_____ IV infusion of D_5NS with 20 mEq KCl

_____ Receiving meperidine via patient-controlled analgesia (PCA)

_____ Nothing by mouth (NPO) status

_____ Telemetry shows atrial fibrillation

➡ - Click on **Laboratory Reports** and review findings.

3. Using the chart below, record Piya Jordan's chemistry results. In the last column, indicate whether values demonstrate an abnormal or normal trend.

Lab Value	Mon 2200	Tues 0630	Wed 0630	Is Trend Normal or Abnormal?
Sodium (Na)				
Potassium (K)				
Chloride (Cl)				
Carbon dioxide (CO_2)				
Blood urea nitrogen (BUN)				

4. The condition indicated by Piya Jordan's potassium levels is known as

_____.

5. Clinical manifestations of the condition identified in the preceding question would include which of the following? Select all that apply.

_____ Confusion

_____ Abnormal ventricular arrhythmias

_____ Flushed skin

_____ Weakness

_____ Thirst

_____ Decreased bowel sounds

_____ Diarrhea

→ • Click on and then review the **History and Physical**.

6. Piya Jordan's BUN is elevated. What is BUN used to measure? What can BUN help to determine? (*Hint:* Refer to your nursing drug guide as needed.)

7. What factors might explain the elevated BUN level that resulted during the preoperative period? What treatment was given that would aid in reversing this condition?

→ • Click on **Return to Nurses' Station**.
 • Click on **403** at the bottom of the screen.
 • Review the Initial Observations.

8. Piya Jordan has IV fluids of _____ running at 100 mL/hour.

9. Piya Jordan's IV solution can best be described as:
 a. isotonic.
 b. hypertonic.
 c. hypotonic.

10. Piya Jordan's IV is running at 100 mL/hour. Assume the IV is being delivered by way of macrodrip tubing. Calculate the drop rate for an IV drop factor of 10 gtt/mL.
 a. 15 gtt/minute
 b. 17 gtt/minute
 c. 19 gtt/minute
 d. 20 gtt/minute

11. Which of the following statements best describes an IV site without complications?
 a. IV infusing at 75 mL/hour, site warm with redness, nontender
 b. IV infusing at 100 mL/hour, site nontender, without redness or swelling
 c. IV infusing at keep-vein-open rate, swelling less than 1 inch around site, cool to touch
 d. IV infusing at 100 mL/hour, pain on palpation over site, skin blanched and cool to touch

→ • Click on **Patient Care** and then on **Physical Assessment**.
 • Complete an assessment of the areas pertaining to Piya Jordan's fluid and electrolyte status by clicking on the body system categories (yellow buttons) and subcategories (green buttons).

12. _____ The findings from the assessment of Piya Jordan's oral mucosa and skin indicate normal hydration and good integrity. (True/False)

→ • Click on **EPR** and then on **Login**.
 • Select **403** from the Patient drop-down menu and **Intake and Output** from the Category drop-down menu.
 • Review the Intake and Output values for Piya Jordan between 2300 on Tuesday and 0700 Wednesday.

13. What is Piya Jordan's fluid balance (intake minus output) for the 8-hour period of 2300 to 0700?

14. Which of the following interventions would be appropriate to manage Piya Jordan's fluid imbalance?
   a. Give oral fluids.
   b. Increase IV infusion rate.
   c. Initiate tube feeding.
   d. Discontinue NG decompression.

Exercise 3

Virtual Hospital Activity

 30 minutes

- Sign in to work at Pacific View Regional Hospital on the Medical-Surgical Floor for Period of Care 1. (*Note:* If you are already in the virtual hospital from a previous exercise, click on **Leave the Floor** and then on **Restart the Program** to get to the sign-in window.)
- From the Patient List, select Patricia Newman (Room 406).
- Click on **Get Report**; review the report and then click on **Go to Nurses' Station**.
- Click on **Chart** and then on **406**.
- Click on and review the **Nursing Admission**.

1. The clinical report summary reveals the following blood gas findings: pH 7.33, PaO_2 70, $PaCO_2$ 47, HCO_3 26, SpO_2 sat 92%.

   a. Do these findings demonstrate acidosis or alkalosis?

   b. Is Patricia Newman's primary physical alteration metabolic or respiratory?

- Click on and review the **History and Physical**.

2. What condition originally caused Patricia Newman to have this alteration in blood gases?
   a. Hypertension
   b. Emphysema
   c. Low flow of oxygen via cannula
   d. Pneumonia

3. Alteration in respiratory function can be caused by three different primary alterations. Which of these apply to the emphysema affecting Patricia Newman?
   a. Hypoventilation
   b. Hyperventilation
   c. Hypoxia
   d. Hypoxemia

4. Patricia Newman's pneumonia complicates her respiratory condition by causing which of the following?
   a. Hypoventilation
   b. Hyperventilation
   c. Hypoxia

 • Click on **Return to Nurses' Station**.
   • Click on **406** at the bottom of the screen.
   • Review the Initial Observations.
   • Click on **Patient Care** and then on **Physical Assessment**.
   • Complete a respiratory assessment by clicking on **Chest** (yellow buttons) and **Back & Spine** (green buttons).

5. Which of the following symptoms is most likely to be the result of respiratory acidosis?
   a. Mild dyspnea
   b. Normal heart sounds
   c. Sinus tachycardia
   d. Coarse crackles

 • Click on **Chart**.
   • Select the chart for Room **406**.
   • Click on and review the **Physician's Orders**.
   • Click on and review **Patient Education**.

6. To better manage the patient's acid-base imbalance, the nurse will attempt to improve Patricia Newman's oxygenation. Match each nursing intervention below with its appropriate rationale.

Nursing Intervention	Rationale
_____ Encourage effective coughing	a. Opens bronchioles to enhance oxygen and carbon dioxide exchange
_____ Instruct patient to perform pursed-lip breathing	b. Relieves hypoxia and helps to minimize dyspnea
_____ Administer bronchodilator by metered-dose inhaler (MDI)	c. Removes secretions that alter diffusion of O_2 and CO_2
_____ Promote fluid intake	d. Reduces thick tenacious secretions that hinder gas diffusion
_____ Administer O_2 at 2 liters by nasal cannula	e. Prevents alveolar collapse, thereby improving O_2 diffusion

LESSON 14

Sleep

 Reading Assignment: Sleep (Chapter 42)

Patients: Pablo Rodriguez, Medical-Surgical Floor, Room 405
William Jefferson, Skilled Nursing Floor, Room 501

Objectives:

1. Identify factors that disrupt sleep.
2. Describe the relationship between disturbed sleep pattern and other nursing diagnoses.
3. Develop a plan of care to promote sleep for a patient.
4. Describe interventions designed to promote sleep.
5. Identify approaches used to evaluate a patient's sleep status.

Exercise 1

Writing Activity

20 minutes

1. _____, _____, _____, and

_____ affect circadian rhythms and daily sleep-wake cycles.

2. During the admission process, a patient reports that he was recently diagnosed with a behaviorally induced circadian rhythm sleep disorder. Based on your knowledge, which of the following factors might be contributing to this disorder?
   a. Restless leg syndrome
   b. Sleepwalking
   c. Narcolepsy
   d. Substance abuse issues

3. A patient is being evaluated for a sleep disorder. The provider has ordered a polysomnogram. Patient teaching should include information about which of the following? Select all that apply.

_____ Electroencephalogram (EEG)

_____ Electromyogram

_____ Holter monitor

_____ Apnea monitor

_____ Electrooculogram (EOG)

4. List the physiologic symptoms associated with sleep deprivation.

5. A patient reports that having a few alcoholic drinks helps him get to sleep. In reality, alcohol has which of the following effects on sleep? Select all that apply.

_____ Reduces rapid eye movement (REM) sleep

_____ Prevents an individual from initially falling asleep

_____ Causes awakening during the night accompanied by difficulty falling back to sleep

_____ Increases sleep apnea

_____ Causes nightmares

6. Identify the concerns associated with long-term use of over-the-counter medications to manage sleep disorders.

7. Vigorous exercise should be avoided within _____ hours of retiring.

Exercise 2

Virtual Hospital Activity

30 minutes

- Sign in to work at Pacific View Regional Hospital on the Medical-Surgical Floor for Period of Care 1. (*Note:* If you are already in the virtual hospital from a previous exercise, click on **Leave the Floor** and then on **Restart the Program** to get to the sign-in window.)
- From the Patient List, select Pablo Rodriguez (Room 405).
- Click on **Get Report**; review the clinical report and then click on **Go to Nurses' Station**.
- Click on **Chart** and then on **405**.
- Click on the **Nursing Admission**, **History and Physical**, and **Physician's Orders**.

1. Why has Pablo Rodriguez been admitted to the hospital?

2. Which of the following factors in Pablo Rodriguez's history are contributing to his sleep problem? Select all that apply.

_____ Eats spicy cheese and refried beans

_____ Smoked heavily until 1 year ago

_____ Depression

_____ Takes celecoxib at home

_____ Pain from subcutaneous nodules

_____ Dyspnea when lying flat

3. Pablo Rodriguez reports "poor sleep and restlessness" upon admission to the hospital. His Nursing Admission notes that he sleeps 6 to 8 hours and then naps 1 to 2 times a day. List three questions to ask to better clarify his sleep pattern.

• Click on **Return to Nurses' Station**.
- Click on **405** at the bottom of the screen.
- Click on **Patient Care** and then on **Nurse-Client Interactions**.
- Select and view the video titled **0730: Symptom Management**. (*Note:* Check the virtual clock to see whether enough time has elapsed. You can use the fast-forward feature to advance the time by 2-minute intervals if the video is not yet available. Then click again on **Patient Care** and on **Nurse-Client Interactions** to refresh the screen.)

Pablo Rodriguez is obviously experiencing emotional distress as a result of his illness. Information from his Nursing Admission further confirms this.

4. _____ Pablo Rodriguez's stress level may be causing him to try too hard to fall asleep. (True/False)

5. _____ Pablo Rodriguez's depressive moods cause the later appearance of REM sleep. (True/False)

6. _____ Depression can cause Pablo Rodriguez to have frequent and early awakening. (True/False)

7. Pablo Rodriguez has the following nursing diagnoses related to his numerous health problems:
   - Impaired Gas Exchange
   - Chronic Pain
   - Disturbed Sleep Pattern
   - Nausea
   What are the interrelationships among these nursing diagnoses?

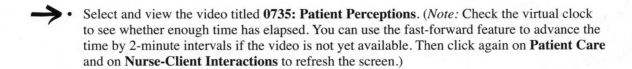 • Select and view the video titled **0735: Patient Perceptions**. (*Note:* Check the virtual clock to see whether enough time has elapsed. You can use the fast-forward feature to advance the time by 2-minute intervals if the video is not yet available. Then click again on **Patient Care** and on **Nurse-Client Interactions** to refresh the screen.)

8. For the nursing diagnosis of Disturbed Sleep Pattern, identify four possible related factors.

9. Pablo Rodriguez's sleep problem is best described as:
   a. sleep apnea.
   b. insomnia.
   c. sleep deprivation.
   d. excessive daytime sleepiness.

Exercise 3

Virtual Hospital Activity

30 minutes

- Sign in to work at Pacific View Regional Hospital on the Skilled Nursing Floor for Period of Care 1. (*Note:* If you are already in the virtual hospital from a previous exercise, click on **Leave the Floor** and then on **Restart the Program** to get to the sign-in window.)
- From the Patient List, select William Jefferson (Room 501).
- Click on **Get Report**; review the report and then click on **Go to Nurses' Station**.
- Click on **Chart** and then on **501**.
- Click on and review the **Nursing Admission**, **History and Physical**, and **Physician's Orders**.

1. Why has William Jefferson been admitted to the Skilled Nursing Floor?

2. William Jefferson's wife reports that her husband seems to have some difficulty with sleeping at home. What food preferences, if eaten in the evening, might be altering his ability to fall asleep? List three.

3. Mrs. Jefferson reports that she does not let her husband nap for more than 1 hour. What would be your response to this information?

→ • Click on and review the **Nursing Admission**.

4. The Nursing Admission notes William Jefferson takes hydrochlorothiazide as part of his normal medication routine. Explain why hydrochlorothiazide might affect a patient's sleep. Does William Jefferson's history confirm such a problem? (*Hint:* Consult the Drug Guide as needed.)

5. William Jefferson is 75 years old. Identify at least four changes in sleep patterns that commonly occur in older adults.

6. _____ Low noises within the extended-care facility, such as staff talking outside of the room, are more likely to arouse William Jefferson from stage 3 sleep. (True/False)

7. _____ If the room is too hot, it can cause William Jefferson to become restless and unable to fall asleep. (True/False)

8. Match each of the following sleep interventions with its corresponding rationale.

Intervention	**Rationale**
_____ Have Mrs. Jefferson offer chamomile tea to her husband in the evening.	a. Promotes maximal ventilation
_____ Recommend that William Jefferson wear loose-fitting sleepwear to bed.	b. Maintains a state of fatigue and promotes relaxation
_____ Recommend a low-running fan in the bedroom at night.	c. Prevents discomfort of full bladder
_____ Encourage the patient and his wife to take their dog for a walk 2 hours before bedtime.	d. Promotes comfort
_____ Always have William Jefferson void before going to bed.	e. Provides a mild sedative effect

9. Discuss possible dietary-related interventions that may help William Jefferson sleep.

Pain Management

 Reading Assignment: Pain Management (Chapter 43)

Patients: Piya Jordan, Medical-Surgical Floor, Room 403
Pablo Rodriguez, Medical-Surgical Floor, Room 405

Objectives:

1. Differentiate between acute and chronic pain.
2. Describe factors that influence pain.
3. Identify presenting signs and symptoms of a patient in pain.
4. Describe cultural implications in pain management.
5. Apply critical thinking in the assessment of a patient in pain.
6. Select appropriate pain relief interventions for two patients.
7. Discuss principles for use of patient-controlled analgesia (PCA).
8. Identify approaches for evaluating a patient's response to pain therapies.

Exercise 1

 Writing Activity

15 minutes

1. The nurse is scheduled to provide care to a patient who would prefer not to take analgesic medications. Identify some nonpharmacologic pain-relief interventions.

2. _____ The use of placebos is considered unethical. (True/False)

3. A nurse is preparing an education program to discuss aging and pain. Which of the following concepts about pain is correct and may be included in the presentation? Select all that apply.

_____ Infants can experience pain.

_____ Pain is a natural part of aging.

_____ Opioids are safe to use in older adults experiencing moderate-to-severe pain.

_____ The onset of a dementia disorder such as Alzheimer's disease reduces the patient's perception of pain.

_____ Older patients make more pain-related complaints.

4. A(n) _____ is the use of medication to enhance the analgesic effectiveness of a prescribed narcotic.

Exercise 2

  Virtual Hospital Activity

30 minutes

- Sign in to work at Pacific View Regional Hospital on the Medical-Surgical Floor for Period of Care 1. (*Note:* If you are already in the virtual hospital from a previous exercise, click on **Leave the Floor** and then on **Restart the Program** to get to the sign-in window.)
- From the Patient List, select Pablo Rodriguez (Room 405).
- Click on **Get Report**; review the report and then click on **Go to Nurses' Station**.
- Click on **Chart** and then on **405**.
- Click on and review the **Nursing Admission** and **History and Physical**.

1. Why has Pablo Rodriguez been admitted to the hospital?

2. Based on data from the Nursing Admission summary, list six different sources of discomfort affecting Pablo Rodriguez.

3. Which of the following best describes the pain of the subcutaneous nodules?
   a. Neuropathic pain
   b. Acute pain
   c. Idiopathic pain
   d. Nociceptive somatic pain

4. _____ Chronic pain from cancer may be sensed at the actual site of the tumor or distant to the site. (True/False)

5. _____ Associated symptoms of chronic pain can include fatigue, anorexia, weight loss, and insomnia. (True/False)

➤ • Click on **Return to Nurses' Station** and then on **405** at the bottom of the screen.
   • Review the Initial Observations.
   • Click on **Patient Care** and then on **Nurse-Client Interactions**.
   • Select and view the video titled **0730: Symptom Management**. (*Note:* Check the virtual clock to see whether enough time has elapsed. You can use the fast-forward feature to advance the time by 2-minute intervals if the video is not yet available. Then click again on **Patient Care** and on **Nurse-Client Interactions** to refresh the screen.)

6. Name two factors, identified in Pablo Rodriguez's admission data, that would increase his perception of pain.

7. Pablo Rodriguez's Hispanic culture influences how he experiences pain and how he is able to express it with family and caregivers. In the nursing history, the patient reported that he wishes the pain to "go away." Based on your observation of the patient during the video, which of the following statements accurately describe factors the nurse should consider in his care? Select all that apply.

   _____ The nurse may need to use probing questions to thoroughly assess Pablo Rodriguez's pain.

   _____ The patient's feelings about the meaning of pain will affect his perception of it.

   _____ Knowing the nature of cancer pain, the nurse should presume how Pablo Rodriguez will respond.

   _____ Whether Pablo Rodriguez is stoic or expressive about pain reflects his Hispanic culture.

   _____ Pablo Rodriguez's language barrier makes it difficult to assess his pain.

→ • Click on **EPR** and then on **Login**.
  • Select **405** from the Patient drop-down menu and **Vital Signs** from the Category drop-down menu. Review the pain assessment for Pablo Rodriguez.

8. Identify the characteristics of pain that are included in the EPR assessment. Select all that apply.

_____ Pain location

_____ Pain intensity

_____ Pain onset

_____ Pain quality

_____ Behavioral effects

_____ Contributing factors

_____ Influence on activities of daily living

→ • Click on **Exit EPR**.
  • Click on **Chart** and then on **405**.
  • Click on **Physician's Orders**. Review the orders for Tuesday at 2300.

9. The EPR data indicated that relieving factors could be referred to in the provider's orders. What is wrong with such an assessment finding?

10. The physician has provided the following order for patient-controlled analgesia: morphine sulfate 0.5 mg IV every 10 min/12 mg in 4-hour lockout. Over a period of 1 hour, what would Pablo Rodriguez's maximum dose be?
   a. 10 mg
   b. 3 mg
   c. 30 mg
   d. 12 mg

11. If, in describing use of the PCA, Pablo Rodriguez said to you, "I am afraid to keep pushing this button so often," what would you say?

• Click on **Return to Room 405**.
  • Click on **MAR**.
  • Review the prescribed medications for Pablo Rodriguez.

12. Match each prescribed medication with its corresponding classification or mechanism of action. (*Hint:* Consult the Drug Guide.)

Medication	**Classification/Mechanism of Action**
_____ Morphine sulfate	a. Antiemetic, blocks serotonin
_____ Metoclopramide hydrochloride	b. Ammonia detoxicant
_____ Neutra-Phos	c. Schedule II narcotic analgesic
_____ Zolpidem	d. Minerals and electrolytes; laxative
_____ Dexamethasone	e. Schedule IV hypnotic
_____ Senna	f. Antiemetic, reduces esophageal reflux
_____ Lactulose	g. Laxative
_____ Ondansetron	h. Corticosteroid

13. Morphine is an opiate. What complications does it cause that could worsen Pablo Rodriguez's current condition?

14. What is the rationale for prescribing two analgesics to manage Pablo Rodriguez's pain?
    a. Providing the IV push medication will reduce his dependence on the PCA pump.
    b. Having multiple analgesic orders will allow the patient to choose which is preferred.
    c. This is standard practice.
    d. Having the two medications provides a means to manage breakthrough pain.

Exercise 3

Virtual Hospital Activity

15 minutes

- Sign in to work at Pacific View Regional Hospital on the Medical-Surgical Floor for Period of Care 2. (*Note:* If you are already in the virtual hospital from a previous exercise, click on **Leave the Floor** and then on **Restart the Program** to get to the sign-in window.)
- From the Patient List, select Pablo Rodriguez (Room 405).
- Click on **Get Report** and then on **Go to Nurses' Station**.
- Click on **Chart** and then on **405**.
- Click on and review the **Nursing Admission**.

1. Pablo Rodriguez's data reveal a number of nursing diagnoses, which are listed below. Match each nursing diagnosis with its defining characteristics from the patient's record. Each nursing diagnosis may have more than one characteristic, and each defining characteristic may apply to more than one nursing diagnosis. (*Hint:* Refer to the NANDA international nursing diagnoses and defining characteristics listings.)

Nursing Diagnoses	**Defining Characteristics**
_____ Nausea	a. Experiencing metallic taste
_____ Chronic Pain	b. Pain reported as 5 on a scale of 0 to 10
_____ Fatigue	c. Reports difficulty falling asleep
_____ Imbalanced Nutrition: Less Than Body Requirements	d. Inability to maintain usual routines
	e. Lost 50 pounds last year
	f. Reports feeling nauseated
	g. Reports feeling weak and tired
	h. Sore, inflamed gums
	i. Loss of appetite

→ • Still in the chart, review the **Patient Education** notes.

2. Explain the purpose for teaching the patient about mouth care.

3. Consider what you know about Pablo Rodriguez. Listed below are nonpharmacologic pain-relief interventions that may or may not be appropriate in helping Pablo Rodriguez obtain pain relief. Provide a rationale to explain why or why not to use each of the therapies for Pablo Rodriguez at this time.

Progressive relaxation

Back rub

Removing pain stimuli

Music

Exercise 4

 Virtual Hospital Activity

 30 minutes

- Sign in to work at Pacific View Regional Hospital on the Medical-Surgical Floor for Period of Care 1. (*Note:* If you are already in the virtual hospital from a previous exercise, click on **Leave the Floor** and then on **Restart the Program** to get to the sign-in window.)
- From the Patient List, select Piya Jordan (Room 403).
- Click on **Get Report** and then on **Go to Nurses' Station**.
- Click on **Chart** and then on **403**.
- Click on and review the **History and Physical**.

   1. After reviewing the History and Physical and the description of Piya Jordan's pain, how would you critique the quality of the physician's pain assessment? Explain.

 - Now review the **Nursing Admission**, specifically the Comfort section near the end of the form.

   2. What characteristics of pain are missing from the Nursing Admission description?

 - Click on **Return to Nurses' Station**.
- Click on **EPR** and **Login**.
- Select **403** from the Patient drop-down menu and **Vital Signs** from the Category drop-down menu.
- Review the pain assessment.
- Click on **Exit EPR**.
- Click on **Patient List**. Access and review Piya Jordan's Clinical Report by clicking on **Get Report** next to her name.

3. Based on the data from the EPR, Piya Jordan is experiencing acute postoperative incisional pain. Her clinical summary reported restlessness and confusion from an overdose of meperidine through her PCA. What would be the priority nursing measure to initiate?
   a. Increase the dosing interval for administration of meperidine.
   b. Initiate more frequent vital signs, including pain assessment.
   c. Reeducate Piya Jordan and her daughter about the proper way to self-administer PCA doses.
   d. Stop the PCA infusion and consult with the physician about changing the drug in the PCA and treating the patient for side effects.

 • Click on **Return to Nurses' Station**.
   • Click on **403** at the bottom of the screen.
   • Review the Initial Observations.
   • Click on **Patient Care** and then on **Nurse-Client Interactions**.
   • Select and view the video titled **0735: Pain—Adverse Drug Event**. (*Note:* Check the virtual clock to see whether enough time has elapsed. You can use the fast-forward feature to advance the time by 2-minute intervals if the video is not yet available. Then click again on **Patient Care** and on **Nurse-Client Interactions** to refresh the screen.)

4. Nonpharmacologic pain-relief interventions can be appropriate for patients in acute pain. What do you know about Piya Jordan that might make nonpharmacologic interventions appealing?

5. The Nursing Admission summary noted that Piya Jordan used a heating pad at home for pain relief. A heating pad provides pain relief through which action?
   a. Biofeedback
   b. Distraction
   c. Reducing pain perception
   d. Cutaneous stimulation

6. Piya Jordan was reported at 0700 to have confusion and restlessness. Would use of a heating pad have been appropriate for pain relief at that time? Explain.

LESSON 16

Nutrition

 Reading Assignment: Nutrition (Chapter 44)

Patients: Jacquline Catanazaro, Medical-Surgical Floor, Room 402
Pablo Rodriguez, Medical-Surgical Floor, Room 405

Objectives:

1. Calculate a patient's body mass index (BMI).
2. Identify the function of select nutrients.
3. Describe factors that place patients at risk for nutritional problems.
4. Conduct a dietary history.
5. Identify clinical signs of nutritional alterations.
6. Identify appropriate diet therapies for patients in the case studies.

Exercise 1

 Writing Activity

🕐 15 minutes

1. The _____ is best defined as
the energy needed to maintain life-sustaining activities for a specific period of time at rest.

2. In a healthy daily diet, fat intake should not exceed what portion of the total intake?
   a. 10%
   b. 15%
   c. 25%
   d. 35%

3. A nurse is caring for a patient who is on aspirin therapy. The nurse correctly recognizes that which of the following will have alterations in absorption rates when combined with aspirin? Select all that apply.

_____ Vitamin B_6

_____ Vitamin B_{12}

_____ Iron

_____ Vitamin C

_____ Vitamin K

4. _____ In certain cultures, menstruation and cancer may be considered cold illnesses requiring the intake of hot foods. (True/False)

5. When caring for a patient receiving enteral feedings, the nurse must assess residual volume with what frequency?
   a. 1 to 2 hours
   b. 2 to 4 hours
   c. 4 to 6 hours
   d. 6 to 8 hours

6. _____ are the most calorie-dense nutrients.

Exercise 2

 Virtual Hospital Activity

 30 minutes

- Sign in to work at Pacific View Regional Hospital on the Medical-Surgical Floor for Period of Care 1. (*Note:* If you are already in the virtual hospital from a previous exercise, click on **Leave the Floor** and then on **Restart the Program** to get to the sign-in window.)
- From the Patient List, select Jacquline Catanazaro (Room 402).
- Click on **Get Report** and then on **Go to Nurses' Station**.
- Click on **Chart** and then on **402**.
- Click on the **Nursing Admission** and **Physician's Orders**. Review the records.

1. Why has Jacquline Catanazaro been admitted to the hospital?

2. Based on your review of the information in the Nursing Admission, complete the following dietary history for Jacquline Catanazaro.

Height

Weight

History of food allergies

Number of meals per day

Food preferences

Food preparation practices

Appetite

History of weight change

Condition of oral cavity

Bowel elimination

3. Calculate Jacquline Catanazaro's BMI. (*Hint:* There are 2.2 pounds in a kilogram; 1 meter equals 39.37 inches.)

$$BMI = \frac{Weight\ (kg)}{Height\ (m)^2}$$

4. Does Jacquline Catanazaro's BMI confirm the admission history report that says the patient is obese?

• Click on **History and Physical**. Review the record.
- Review **Consultations**, specifically the Psychiatric Consult.

5. Which of the following factors most likely has contributed to Jacquline Catanazaro's loss of appetite for the last week? Select all that apply.

_____ Albuterol

_____ Anxiety

_____ Loxapine

_____ Shortness of breath

_____ Excessive sleep

6. According to MyPlate, which food should represent the greater part of the diet?
   a. Fruits
   b. Vegetables
   c. Grains
   d. Proteins

• Click on **Physician's Orders**.

7. The physician has ordered a(n) _____ diet for Jacquline Catanazaro.

8. Jacquline Catanazaro's constipation might be relieved by an increase in fruits, vegetables,

and _____.

9. Review Jacquline Catanazaro's prescribed medications. Which of the following medications may result in an increase in appetite? (*Hint:* See Table 44-2 in your textbook.)
   a. Albuterol
   b. Prednisone
   c. Amoxicillin
   d. Beclomethasone
   e. Ipratropium bromide

10. What would be an appropriate approach for assessing Jacquline Catanazaro's nutritional intake once she is discharged?

11. Based on your review of the medical record, list three interventions you might use to improve Jacquline Catanazaro's nutritional status.

Exercise 3

Virtual Hospital Activity

30 minutes

- Sign in to work at Pacific View Regional Hospital on the Medical-Surgical Floor for Period of Care 2. (*Note:* If you are already in the virtual hospital from a previous exercise, click on **Leave the Floor** and then on **Restart the Program** to get to the sign-in window.)
- From the Patient List, select Pablo Rodriguez (Room 405).
- Click on **Get Report** and then on **Go to Nurses' Station**.
- Click on **Chart** and then on **405**.
- Click on the **Nursing Admission** and **History and Physical**. Review the records.

1. Why has Pablo Rodriguez been admitted to the hospital?

2. List three factors that may contribute to Pablo Rodriguez's loss of appetite.

3. What impact does radiation therapy have on the gastrointestinal system?

4. Below, match each nursing diagnosis with its cluster of defining characteristics.

Nursing Diagnosis	**Defining Characteristics**
_____ Nausea	a. Sore buccal cavity, aversion to eating, body weight 20% below ideal, poor muscle tone
_____ Imbalanced Nutrition: Less Than Body Requirements	b. Metallic taste, aversion to food, reports feeling of nausea
_____ Chronic Pain	c. Weight change, changes in sleep pattern, fatigue, loss of appetite

5. Pablo Rodriguez has received chemotherapy and radiation, both of which can affect a patient's immune system. His loss of 50 pounds over a year and his current symptoms indicate malnutrition. Malnutrition can cause which of the following?
   a. Increased skin density
   b. Shorter time for activation of lymphocytes
   c. Reduced antibodies
   d. Increased T cell formation

6. Based on your chart review, which of the following physical findings could be related to Pablo Rodriguez's nutritional status? Select all that apply.

   _____ Mild swelling of lower extremities

   _____ Skin warm and dry

   _____ No accessory muscle use

   _____ Swollen red gums

   _____ Capillary refill greater than 4 seconds

   _____ General muscle weakness

LESSON 17

Elimination

Reading Assignment: Urinary Elimination (Chapter 45)
Bowel Elimination (Chapter 46)

Patients: Jacquline Catanazaro, Medical-Surgical Floor, Room 402
Piya Jordan, Medical-Surgical Floor, Room 403

Objectives:

1. Describe factors that influence normal defecation and urination.
2. Develop a plan of care for a patient with a bowel elimination alteration.
3. Identify nursing interventions used to manage bowel elimination problems.
4. Describe principles used in the care of an indwelling urinary catheter.
5. Describe nursing interventions designed to reduce the risk for urinary tract infection.

Exercise 1

Writing Activity

30 minutes

1. The kidneys are responsible for the production of _____ to maintain normal red blood cell volume.

2. Identify factors that influence urination.

3. Below, match each term with the corresponding definition.

Term	Definition
_____ Micturition	a. Difficult or painful urination
_____ Dysuria	b. Involuntary urination that occurs during sleep
_____ Oliguria	c. Diminished, scant amounts of urine
_____ Anuria	d. The process of emptying the bladder
_____ Polyuria	e. The absence of urine
_____ Enuresis	f. The production of an excess of urine
_____ Nocturia	g. Urination at nighttime
_____ Hematuria	h. Blood in the urine

4. _____ measures the concentration of particles in urine.

5. _____ When using the French measuring system for catheters, the larger the gauge number, the larger the catheter size. (True/False)

6. Below, match each term with the corresponding definition.

Term	Definition
_____ Feces	a. The process by which feces and flatus pass through the rectum and anal canal
_____ Peristalsis	b. Body waste discharged from the intestine
_____ Flatus	c. Collection of hardened feces in the rectum or sigmoid colon preventing passage of a normal stool
_____ Defecation	d. A condition in which feces are abnormally hard and dry
_____ Valsalva maneuver	e. Rhythmic smooth muscle contractions that propel stool through the intestines
_____ Constipation	f. Rapid movement of fecal matter through the intestine resulting in diminished absorption of water, nutrients, and electrolytes
_____ Fecal impaction	g. Swallowed air and gases produced through the digestive process
_____ Diarrhea	h. A voluntary contraction of the abdominal muscles while maintaining forced expiration against a closed airway

7. A patient passes a clay-colored stool. Based on your knowledge, you recognize that a potential cause of the clay-colored stool is:
   a. iron deficient anemia.
   b. fat malabsorption disorder.
   c. absence of bile.
   d. excessive fat in the stool.

8. A patient at average risk for the development of colorectal cancer should have an initial colonoscopy at age:
   a. 35 years.
   b. 40 years.
   c. 45 years.
   d. 50 years.

Exercise 2

 Virtual Hospital Activity

 45 minutes

- Sign in to work at Pacific View Regional Hospital on the Medical-Surgical Floor for Period of Care 1. (*Note:* If you are already in the virtual hospital from a previous exercise, click on **Leave the Floor** and then on **Restart the Program** to get to the sign-in window.)
- From the Patient List, select Piya Jordan (Room 403).
- Click on **Get Report**; review the report and then click on **Go to Nurses' Station**.
- Click on **Chart** and then on **403**.
- Click on and review the **History and Physical**.
- Click on **Diagnostic Reports** and review the summary of abdominal CT.
- Click on and review the **Physician's Notes**.

1. What is Piya Jordan's medical diagnosis?

2. Piya Jordan's History & Physical reports ribbonlike stool and the presence of blood in her stool. Explain the source of these symptoms.

3. Based on your review of the abdominal CT summary, removal of Piya Jordan's mass would likely cause what change in her elimination in the future? Explain.

→ • Click on and review the **Nursing Admission**.

4. Below, match each factor with the corresponding effect on bowel elimination.

Factor	Effect on Bowel Elimination
_____ Physical activity	a. Increases peristalsis
_____ Fluid intake less than 1000 mL daily	b. Decreases peristalsis
_____ High-fiber diet	c. Suppresses defecation
_____ Older adulthood	
_____ Pain	
_____ Lactose intolerance	

5. Based on your knowledge that Piya Jordan has had a colon resection, as well as your review of her elimination history, list three recommendations you would make to ensure normal bowel elimination once she goes home.

→ • Still in the chart, review the **Physician's Orders** and the **Laboratory Reports**.

6. Piya Jordan has had a urinalysis ordered for which of the following reasons?
   a. It is needed as a preoperative screening.
   b. Her intravenous (IV) infusion contains potassium.
   c. Her past history of diabetes mellitus suggests there may be glucose in her urine.
   d. She is at risk for infection because of the presence of the urinary catheter.

7. Piya Jordan's specific gravity value was elevated. To what can this be attributed?

8. Which of the following catheter types is being used by Piya Jordan?
   a. Texas
   b. Straight
   c. Condom
   d. Foley
   e. Irrigation
   f. Suprapubic

9. Piya Jordan has a urinary catheter in place. Using the diagram below, identify potential sites through which infectious organisms may be introduced into a urinary drainage system. List the letters associated with any areas of concern.

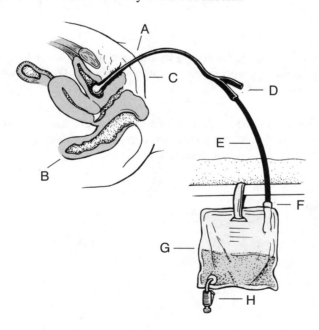

• Click on **Return to Nurses' Station**.
- Click on **403** at the bottom of the screen.
- Review the Initial Observations.
- Click on **Patient Care** and then on **Physical Assessment**.

10. In the left column below, list the physical assessment categories for which you would choose to perform a focused assessment of the function and effects of Piya Jordan's urinary catheter. For each category, provide a rationale for your selection.

Categories to Assess	Rationale

 • Based on your answers to the previous question, perform the focused assessment on Piya Jordan by clicking on the appropriate body system categories (yellow buttons) and subcategories (green buttons).

11. Based on your assessment of Piya Jordan's catheter and drainage system, was the catheter and drainage system anchored and positioned correctly? Explain. (*Hint:* Refer to the photo presented as part of the Urologic assessment data.)

Exercise 3

Virtual Hospital Activity

20 minutes

- Sign in to work at Pacific View Regional Hospital on the Medical-Surgical Floor for Period of Care 2. (*Note:* If you are already in the virtual hospital from a previous exercise, click on **Leave the Floor** and then on **Restart the Program** to get to the sign-in window.)
- From the Patient List, select Jacquline Catanazaro (Room 402).
- Click on **Get Report**; review the report and then click on **Go to Nurses' Station**.
- Click on **Chart** and then on **402**.
- Click on **Nursing Admission** and review the record.

1. Jacquline Catanazaro was admitted for exacerbation of asthma. The Nursing Admission indicates a patient-reported bowel movement of every 1 to 2 days, a perception of constipation, and a hard stool. What two additional symptoms might you assess to confirm constipation for this patient?

2. Which of the following factors contribute to Jacquline Catanazaro's bowel elimination problems? Select all that apply.

_____ Physical inactivity

_____ Age

_____ Emotional stress

_____ Limited intake of high-fiber foods

_____ Reduced fluid intake

_____ Obesity

 - Click on **Return to Nurses' Station**.
- Click on **402** at the bottom of the screen.
- Review the Initial Observations.
- Click on **Patient Care** and then on **Physical Assessment**.
- Click on **Abdomen** (yellow buttons) and review the examination of the abdomen by clicking on the available body system subcategories (green buttons).

3. The findings listed below were assessed during Jacquline Catanazaro's abdominal assessment. Next to each finding, describe what you would be more likely to find if the patient had constipation.

Actual Physical Finding	Likely Finding If Patient Had Constipation
Abdomen soft and flat	
Bowel sounds normal	
No abdominal tenderness or masses	

- Click on **Patient Care** and then on **Nurse-Client Interactions**.
- Select and view the video titled **1140: Compliance—Medications**. (*Note:* Check the virtual clock to see whether enough time has elapsed. You can use the fast-forward feature to advance the time by 2-minute intervals if the video is not yet available. Then click again on **Patient Care** and on **Nurse-Client Interactions** to refresh the screen.)

4. Jacquline Catanazaro's Nursing Admission and the video reveal the following three data clusters. Identify the nursing diagnosis for each cluster. (*Hint:* Refer to a resource for NANDA nursing diagnoses.)

Data Cluster 1	Nursing Diagnosis
Emotional stress	
Insufficient fiber intake	
Poor eating habits; does not eat vegetables or fruits	
Insufficient fluid intake	
Antipsychotic/sedative use	

Data Cluster 2	Nursing Diagnosis
Dysfunctional eating pattern; eats 4 to 6 meals a day	
Sedentary activity level	
Weight 20% above ideal for height	

Data Cluster 3	Nursing Diagnosis
Inability to take responsibility for meeting health practices; does not remember to take medications	
Lack of adaptive behavior to environmental changes; anxious and agitated	
Lack of knowledge regarding health practices; states, "It takes a lot for me to remember"	

5. Assume that the nurse caring for Jacquline Catanazaro decided to consult with the physician about ordering a medication for the patient. What might be the best recommendation to relieve her constipation? Explain.

6. Review Jacquline Catanazaro's prescribed medications. Which of the medications are associated with constipation? Select all that apply. (*Hint:* Refer to the Drug Guide as needed.)

_____ Beclomethasone metered-dose inhaler (MDI)

_____ Ipratropium bromide MDI

_____ Amoxicillin

_____ Prednisone

_____ Albuterol MDI

_____ Ziprasidone

_____ Ibuprofen

7. If you were the nurse caring for Jacquline Catanazaro 2 days after initiating treatment for constipation, what evaluation measures would you use to determine whether the plan of care was effective?

LESSON # 18

Care of the Surgical Patient

Reading Assignment: Skin Integrity and Wound Care (Chapter 48)
Care of Surgical Patients (Chapter 50)

Patient: Piya Jordan, Medical-Surgical Floor, Room 403

Objectives:

1. Describe criteria to use in the preoperative assessment of a surgical patient.
2. Explain the rationale for postoperative exercises.
3. Discuss principles to incorporate in a preoperative teaching plan.
4. Describe a patient's risks for postoperative complications.
5. Identify risks associated with different forms of anesthesia.
6. Apply critical thinking to the assessment of a postoperative patient.
7. Identify signs and symptoms of common postoperative complications.
8. Describe nursing interventions for preventing postoperative complications.

Exercise 1

Writing Activity

  15 minutes

1. Below, match each type of surgery with the corresponding definition.

Type of Surgery	Definition
_____ Urgent	a. Performed to restore function that was lost or reduced as a result of congenital anomalies
_____ Diagnostic	
_____ Palliative	b. Necessary for patient's health; may prevent additional problems from developing
_____ Constructive	c. Excision or removal of a diseased body part
_____ Ablative	d. Exploration allowing for the confirmation of a diagnosis
	e. Performed to reduce intensity of disease symptoms

2. A patient reports taking large doses of ibuprofen during the preoperative period. Which of the following complications is the patient at an increased risk for developing?
   a. Increased bleeding
   b. Postoperative infection
   c. Electrolyte imbalance
   d. Hypotension

3. After surgery, it is recommended that the patient have at least _____ kcal/day for nutritional maintenance.

4. _____ Antiembolic stockings must be worn around the clock during the first 2 days of the postoperative experience. (True/False)

5. _____ anesthesia involves loss of sensation to a specific body site.

6. Surgeries requiring extensive invasion and manipulation of the body require

   _____ anesthesia.

7. During the postoperative period, urinary output less than _____ warrants contacting the physician.
   a. 100 mL/hour
   b. 75 mL/hour
   c. 50 mL/hour
   d. 30 mL/hour

8. Handling of the bowel during surgery may result in a nonmechanical obstruction known as

   a(n) _____.

9. A nurse is planning education for a patient who has just had abdominal surgery. The nurse should recommend the practice of diaphragmatic breathing exercises with what frequency while the patient is awake?
   a. Every hour
   b. Every 2 hours
   c. Every 4 hours
   d. Every 6 to 8 hours

Exercise 2

  Virtual Hospital Activity

45 minutes

- Sign in to work at Pacific View Regional Hospital on the Medical-Surgical Floor for Period of Care 1. (*Note:* If you are already in the virtual hospital from a previous exercise, click on **Leave the Floor** and then on **Restart the Program** to get to the sign-in window.)
- From the Patient List, select Piya Jordan (Room 403).
- Click on **Get Report**; review the report and then click on **Go to Nurses' Station**.
- Click on **Chart** and then on **403**.
- Click on and review the **Nursing Admission**.

1. Review and discuss the factors that led Piya Jordan to undergo surgery.

2. Based on the Nursing Admission data, choose the surgical risk factors that apply to Piya Jordan. Select all that apply.

   _____ Obesity

   _____ Heart disease

   _____ Fever

   _____ Nutritional imbalance

   _____ Chronic pain

   _____ Age

   _____ Liver disease

3. Identify two alterations of the cardiovascular system that may apply to Piya Jordan because of her age.

→ • Click on and then review the **History and Physical** and **Laboratory Results**.

4. The History and Physical noted the need to correct Piya Jordan's electrolytes and reverse anticoagulation before surgery. Which preoperative laboratory values were abnormal in Piya Jordan's case? Select all that apply.

_____ Red blood cell count (RBC)

_____ International normalized ratio (INR)

_____ Potassium (K^+)

_____ Sodium (Na)

_____ Hemoglobin (Hgb)

_____ Creatinine

5. Why do you think Piya Jordan's Hgb and RBC values were lower than normal before surgery? Why are changes in these lab values significant?

6. What is the most likely reason that Piya Jordan's INR is higher than normal?
   a. Inflammation of her knee joints
   b. Warfarin therapy at home
   c. Irregular nature of her heart rate
   d. Blood in her stool

7. Because of the elevated INR, Piya Jordan would be at risk for which of the following complications during surgery?
   a. Urinary retention
   b. Pneumonia
   c. Paralytic ileus
   d. Hemorrhage

 • Still in the chart, click again on **Nursing Admission** and review the summaries for Perception and Cognition, Self-Perception, Role Relationships, and Coping and Stress Tolerance.

• Now review the **Nurse's Notes** from Tuesday 0330 to Tuesday 0900.

8. The nurse's assessment should identify factors that will have an affect on the patient's ability to receive and understand preoperative instruction. Listed below are numerous factors identified in Piya Jordan's assessment. Complete this exercise by indicating whether each factor would facilitate instruction (positive effect) or would be a barrier to instruction (negative effect).

Assessment Factor	Effect on Instruction
_____ Patient reports a pain score of 8 out of 10.	a. Positive
_____ Patient expresses being anxious about husband's welfare.	b. Negative
_____ Daughter is supportive of mother.	
_____ Patient is fearful of cancer diagnosis.	
_____ Patient speaks English and has a college education.	
_____ Patient reports feeling nauseated.	

9. Based on information from the Nurse's Notes and Nursing Admission, what would be the best time to teach Piya Jordan about deep breathing and coughing exercises? Give a rationale.

10. After surgery, it is important to turn patients frequently. What factor in Piya Jordan's history might make turning difficult for her?

Exercise 3

Virtual Hospital Activity

30 minutes

- Sign in to work at Pacific View Regional Hospital on the Medical-Surgical Floor for Period of Care 1. (*Note:* If you are already in the virtual hospital from a previous exercise, click on **Leave the Floor** and then on **Restart the Program** to get to the sign-in window.)
- From the Patient List, select Piya Jordan (Room 403).
- Click on **Get Report**; and then on **Go to Nurses' Station**.
- Click on **Chart** and then on **403**.
- Click on and review the **Nurse's Notes**, **Surgical Reports**, and **Physician's Notes**.

1. For each of the interventions listed below, give a rationale for its use in Piya Jordan's case.

Jackson-Pratt drain

Sequential compression device (SCD)

Nasogastric (NG) tube

Abdominal dressing

2. Based on your review of the clinical summary and the Nurse's Notes, for what common postoperative complication might Piya Jordan be at risk, unless the nurse more actively intervenes? Give a rationale and explain the interventions required.

 • Click on **Return to Nurses' Station**.
   • Click on **403** at the bottom of the screen.
   • Click on **Patient Care** and then on **Physical Assessment**.
   • Click on **Abdomen** (yellow buttons) and review the findings of the abdominal assessment, specifically the subcategories of **Integumentary** and **Gastrointestinal** (green buttons).

3. What type of dressing does Piya Jordan have over her abdomen? How is it secured?

4. Which of the following best describes the type of healing that will result with Piya Jordan's surgical wound?
   a. Primary intention
   b. Secondary intention
   c. Tertiary intention

5. What is the most critical time for healing of a surgical wound?
   a. First 24 hours postoperative
   b. 7 days postoperative
   c. 24 to 72 hours postoperative
   d. 15 to 20 days postoperative

6. As the nurse caring for Piya Jordan postoperatively, you would want to do a focused assessment when you begin your care. On which assessment categories would you choose to focus postoperatively? (*Hint:* Do not forget to assess equipment.)

 • When you have completed your focused assessment, click on **Leave the Floor**.
• From the Floor Menu, choose **Look at Your Preceptor's Evaluation**.
• Next, click on **Examination Report** to see how you did.

Exercise 4

 Virtual Hospital Activity

 30 minutes

• Sign in to work at Pacific View Regional Hospital on the Medical-Surgical Floor for Period of Care 2. (*Note:* If you are already in the virtual hospital from a previous exercise, click on **Leave the Floor** and then on **Restart the Program** to get to the sign-in window.)
• From the Patient List, select Piya Jordan (Room 403).
• Click on **Get Report**; review the report and then click on **Go to Nurses' Station**.
• Click on **Chart** and then on **403**.
• Click on and review the **Nursing Admission** and the **Surgical Reports**.

 1. Review the data from the PACU discharge flow sheet. Compare the data with the Modified Aldrete Score in your textbook. What score would you give Piya Jordan when she left the PACU? (*Hint:* See Table 50-7 in your textbook.)

2. Take into consideration the type of anesthesia that Piya Jordan received preoperatively. Which complication is she is at risk for developing as a result of the type of anesthesia she received?
   a. Respiratory depression, cardiovascular irritability, and liver damage
   b. Respiratory paralysis and hypotension
   c. Loss of sensation and pain reception in operative area
   d. Headache, urinary retention, and back pain

→ • Click on **Nurse's Notes** and review the notes for Wednesday at 1115.
  • Click on **Return to Nurses' Station**.
  • Click on **403** at the bottom of the screen.
  • Review the Initial Observations.
  • Click on **Patient Care** and then on **Nurse-Client Interactions**.
  • Select and view the video titled **1115: Interventions—Nausea, Blood**. (*Note:* Check the virtual clock to see whether enough time has elapsed. You can use the fast-forward feature to advance the time by 2-minute intervals if the video is not yet available. Then click again on **Patient Care** and on **Nurse-Client Interactions** to refresh the screen.)

3. Piya Jordan is complaining of nausea. What is the likely source of the nausea?

4. Identify three assessments necessary to determine the source and nature of Piya Jordan's nausea.

5. If patency of Piya Jordan's NG tube is in question, what is the appropriate action for the nurse to take?
   a. Remove the tube from suction and call the physician.
   b. Irrigate the tube with normal saline.
   c. Reposition the tube.
   d. Obtain an x-ray of the abdomen.

→ • Click on **Physical Assessment**.
  • Click on **Chest** (yellow buttons) and then on the appropriate subcategories (green buttons) to complete a focused assessment of Piya Jordan's chest.
  • Click on **Abdomen** and the related subcategories to review the abdominal assessment.
  • Click on **Take Vital Signs** at the top of the screen.

6. In reviewing the data available for Piya Jordan, clusters of data are revealed from the assessment. One data cluster for this patient is listed below:
   - Chest expansion decreased
   - Decreased aeration, both lower lobes
   - Has had acute pain
   - Abdomen tender to palpation
   - Has not used incentive spirometer

   What potential problem/nursing diagnosis is indicated by this data cluster?

7. A nurse who has cared for Piya Jordan tells you that one of her nursing diagnoses is Risk for Infection. Give a rationale for why this diagnosis would apply to Piya Jordan.

8. Complete the plan of care below for the nursing diagnosis Ineffective Breathing Pattern.

Nursing Diagnosis: Ineffective Breathing Pattern

Goal

Expected Outcomes

Interventions

1.

2.

3.

4.

Evaluation Measures

1.

2.

3.

Wound Care

 Reading Assignment: Skin Integrity and Wound Care (Chapter 48)

Patients: Harry George, Medical-Surgical Floor, Room 401
Goro Oishi, Skilled Nursing Floor, Room 505

Objectives:

1. Describe risk factors contributing to the formation of pressure ulcers.
2. Use a pressure ulcer risk assessment tool for a patient.
3. Explain factors that slow or promote wound healing.
4. Describe characteristics of a wound.
5. Identify interventions used to prevent the formation of pressure ulcers.
6. Explain the purpose of a wound dressing.
7. Discuss factors to consider when selecting a wound dressing.

Exercise 1

 Writing Activity

10 minutes

1. List at least three nursing actions that are important when preparing a patient for a dressing change.

2. _____ Hydrocolloid dressings support wound healing by debriding necrotic wounds. (True/False)

3. _____ Hydrogel dressings can absorb large amounts of exudate. (True/False)

4. _____ Before removing a wet-to-dry dressing, you should moisten the dressing with saline. (True/False)

5. _____ When selecting a dressing, you should choose one that keeps the surrounding intact skin dry. (True/False)

6. When completing the assessment of a pressure ulcer, you note the presence of yellow exudate. The ulceration extends into the subcutaneous tissue. Which stage of ulcer does this represent?
   a. Stage I
   b. Stage II
   c. Stage III
   d. Stage IV

7. A patient is planning to increase zinc intake to promote wound healing. Which of the following foods should be included in the diet to address this plan?
   a. Eggs
   b. Oranges
   c. Broccoli
   d. Fish
   e. Potatoes

8. A pressure ulcer has the presence of stringy tissue attached to the wound bed. Which of the following terms may be used to correctly describe this manifestation?
   a. Eschar
   b. Slough
   c. Pus
   d. Granulation tissue

Exercise 2

 Virtual Hospital Activity

 20 minutes

- Sign in to work at Pacific View Regional Hospital on the Medical-Surgical Floor for Period of Care 1. (*Note:* If you are already in the virtual hospital from a previous exercise, click on **Leave the Floor** and then on **Restart the Program** to get to the sign-in window.)
- From the Patient List, select Harry George (Room 401).
- Click on **Get Report**; read the report and then click on **Go to Nurses' Station**.
- Click on **Chart** and then on **401**.
- Click on and review the **Nursing Admission** and **History and Physical**.

1. Why has Harry George been admitted to the hospital?

2. Listed below are factors that influence wound healing. Which factors apply to Harry George? Select all that apply.

_____ Nutrition

_____ Smoking

_____ Circulation

_____ Drugs

_____ Obesity

_____ Infection

_____ Age

_____ Wound stress

_____ Diabetes

→ • Click on **Return to Nurses' Station**.
  • Click on **401** at the bottom of the screen.
  • Read the Initial Observations.

3. Explain why Harry George's left foot is elevated.

→ • Click on **Patient Care** and then on **Physical Assessment**.
  • Click on **Lower Extremities** (yellow buttons) and review each of the four subcategories (green buttons) for assessment findings.

4. Based on the description of Harry George's wound, the type of drainage present can best be described as:
   a. thick, yellow, or brown.
   b. clear, watery plasma.
   c. pale, red, watery.
   d. bright red.

• Click on **Chart** and then on **401**.
 • Click on **History and Physical** and review the Social History section.

5. What factor(s) in Harry George's social history may be implicated in his ability to care for his wound? Explain.

 • Click on and then review the **Physician's Notes**.
 • Click on **Consultations** and review the Wound Care Team Consult.

6. The wound care note describes Harry George's dressing as occlusive. Which of the following dressings is most likely being used for Harry George?
   a. Wet to dry
   b. Telfa gauze
   c. Hydrocolloid
   d. Foam dressing

7. Give a rationale for your answer to the previous question.

Exercise 3

 Virtual Hospital Activity

45 minutes

 • Sign in to work at Pacific View Regional Hospital on the Skilled Nursing Floor for Period of Care 1. (*Note:* If you are already in the virtual hospital from a previous exercise, click on **Leave the Floor** and then on **Restart the Program** to get to the sign-in window.)
 • From the Patient List, select Goro Oishi (Room 505).
 • Click on **Get Report**; review the report and then click on **Go to Nurses' Station**.
 • Click on **Chart** and then on **505**.
 • Click on and review the **Nursing Admission** and **History and Physical**.

1. Which of the following risk factors are currently placing Goro Oishi at risk for developing a pressure ulcer? Select all that apply.

_____ Impaired sensation

_____ Impaired mobility

_____ Altered level of consciousness

_____ Moisture

 2. Using the Braden Scale, determine Goro Oishi's risk for developing pressure ulcers. Explain the process by which you arrived at your conclusion and specify the patient's Braden Scale score. (*Hint:* See Table 48-3 in your textbook.)

3. What intervention is most likely preventing prolonged exposure of Goro Oishi's skin to moisture?

 • Click on **Return to Nurses' Station**.
• Click on **505** at the bottom of the screen.
• Review the Initial Observations.
• Click on **Patient Care** and then on **Physical Assessment**.
• Click on **Head & Neck** and then on **Integumentary**; then review the findings. Complete an assessment of the integumentary system by clicking on each of the remaining six body system categories (yellow buttons) and clicking on **Integumentary** within each category.

4. For which of the locations identified below is Goro Oishi at risk for developing a pressure ulcer?

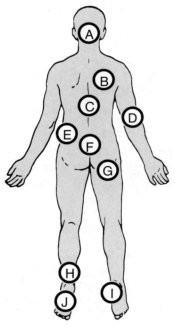

- Click on **EPR** and then on **Login**.
- Select **505** from the Patient drop-down menu and **Integumentary** from the Category drop-down menu. Review the data.
- Select **Hygiene and Comfort** from the Category drop-down menu and review the data.

5. Goro Oishi's Braden Scale score indicates that he is at high risk for developing a pressure ulcer. List at least three interventions for a high-risk ulcer prevention protocol.

6. Answer the following questions based on your review of Goro Oishi's EPR data.

   a. Do you believe Goro Oishi is being turned often enough? Explain.

   b. At what time is he due to be turned again, according to the current schedule?

   c. In what position should he next be placed?

   d. What specialty mattress is currently in use?

7. Which of the following are appropriate interventions for the nurse to perform each time Goro Oishi is turned? Select all that apply.

   _____   Assess the area on which the patient was previously lying for redness.

   _____   Massage any area of redness.

   _____   Check underlying linen for moisture.

   _____   Apply additional moisturizer to the skin.

8. If you were selecting a support surface on which to place Goro Oishi, what type would you choose? Give a rationale.

• Click on **Exit EPR**.
- Click on **Chart** and then on **505**.
- Review the **Nurse's Notes**.

9. Goro Oishi is currently receiving IV fluids. What benefit will the ordered change in nutritional therapy provide for the patient?